Y0-EFE-882

D1712053

GOLDEN INDEPENDENCE

A CAREGIVER'S PRACTICAL GUIDE TO HEALTH AND
SAFETY FOR INDIVIDUALS DURING THEIR GOLDEN YEARS.

PAULA E. GIBESON

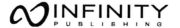

INFINITY PUBLISHING
1094 New DeHaven Street, Suite 100
West Conshohocken, PA 19428-2713
Toll-free (877) BUY BOOK
Local Phone (610) 941-9999
Fax (610) 941-9959
Info@buybooksontheweb.com
www.buybooksontheweb.com

INTRODUCTION

I believe the saying is true, "there's no place like home." People know where everything is located. The familiarity of one's own house provides a safe and secure feeling. Memories abound from every room. There's just no other place like it.

As people age, the desire to live in their own home for the rest of their lives translates into determination to stay independent. What individuals may not realize is that sometimes there may be levels of assistance that promote the safety necessary for them to be able to remain in their beloved house.

There are three sections of this book to help guide individuals and their caregivers. Section 1 discusses issues that affect the quality of life. Section 2 addresses challenging behaviors. Although this is not intended to be a mental health resource, it can be very helpful for caregivers to know how to adapt to their loved ones conduct. Section 3 explains safety in each part of the house.

The ultimate goal is to convey an appreciation of the golden years of a person's life. It is the desire to promote independence with all due respect to safety. By compromising health issues, an elderly individual may not realize they are jeopardizing their independence. The information in *Golden Independence* provides an opportunity to balance all individual considerations with options for seniors and their caregivers.

DISCLAIMER

The information offered in this book is not intended to be medical advice or replace the directions of direct health care providers. The descriptions are presented to ease caregiver stress and provide ideas to promote safety for senior citizens.

Please note, everyone needs to have their own primary health care provider. That professional should be aware of all of the health and safety concerns of their patients. It is recommended to always abide by their health care provider's directions.

Examples have been used at times to assist in understanding situations. However, all characters depicted in this book are fictitious for the purpose of displaying a typical setting or occurrence. Any similarities to an actual individual are entirely coincidental.

This book is dedicated to my two favorite teachers,
Myra and Richard Gibeson,
lovingly known as Mom and Dad.

TABLE OF CONTENTS

SECTION 3: A WALK THROUGH THE HOUSE.......179

SECTION 1

QUALITY OF LIFE

During thirty years of providing nursing care for people over sixty years old, I learned many practical ways to promote health care for specific issues. By covering a range of subjects from falls to incontinence, I want to share thoughts and suggestions to assist individuals and caregivers to achieve and maintain safe independence in everyday living.

Each chapter provides a thought to consider, why the topic for that chapter is significant, goals, interventions, and what to anticipate. People frequently wonder when it is appropriate to contact their health care provider. How to discuss issues of concern productively with health care personnel is also an integral part of each chapter.

One of my priorities as a nurse was to always remember that the individual in front of me deserved respect no matter what their current cognitive or physical challenges were. With that perspective, I offer my professional experience and knowledge for the purpose of offering caregivers information about how to care for others with dignity as a priority.

Chapter 1

THE TOPIC . . . . BATHING

The Reason for the Topic:

- **Routine bathing promotes healthy skin and prevents infections.**
- **Cleanliness helps people to feel better and potentially more relaxed.**
- **Avoiding a foul odor is socially beneficial.**

Just a thought:

In the early years of my career, I worked as a nursing assistant in a long term care unit. In those days, principles of patient's rights were not discussed.

As I think about some the individuals who would demonstrate their objections to bathing, I can't help but wonder how differently things could have been handled.

Today with individual preferences as a priority, I now realize the importance of learning personal choices. Offering the time of day that a person has always bathed can be helpful. Listening to fears and anxieties related to bathing can prevent recurrent struggles. What is it about bathing that caregivers need to know to make the whole process a smooth experience for the individual?

Bath time is easier for the caregiver when the recipient participates with a positive anticipation.

Goals:

- Clean skin with no areas of breakdown, infection, rashes, or odor.
- A positive experience for the recipient.

Interventions:

- Routine bathing two to three times a week.
- Observe skin for rashes or potential areas of infection or skin breakdown.
- Take extra care to clean skin folds as there is an increased likelihood of cracks and infections.
    - o This includes areas such as under the breasts, groin area, buttocks, etc.
    - o Be sure to cleanse the skin between the skin folds. Rinse thoroughly, and dry.
    - o Place a plain white soft cloth between the folds to prevent perspiration from causing redness, cracks, and infections.
    - o Remember bacteria are more likely to grow in a dark, damp, warm environment. Bacteria may cause skin breakdown, infection, and odor.
- If rashes appear after bathing it may be due to inadequate rinsing or an allergy to the soap.
    - o If there appears to be an allergy to the soap, try using a hypoallergenic soap.
- For people who are incontinent it is especially important to cleanse and dry the peri area.
    - o Sometimes it is difficult to be sure this area is adequately rinsed. Try to use a rinse free peri wash.
    - o This also allows for cleansing the skin after each episode of incontinence.
- Do not use powder after bathing. Powder can clog pores.
    - o Consider using lotion instead of powder to maintain skin hydration.

- Always be sure to dry between the toes to prevent cracks in the skin.
- There can be a number of reasons why people choose to avoid bathing.
  - o Those issues are addressed in the behavior section under Problem Behaviors, Chapter 34.

Possible outcomes:
- An adverse outcome would be lack of adequate bathing which results in body odor, infections, and skin breakdown.
- A positive outcome includes routine bathing with clean odor free skin.
- Hopefully, bath time itself is a positive experience.

When to Call for Assistance:
- If there are skin areas that have rashes, skin breakdown, or infection, consider requesting a dermatologist consult.

What the Doctor needs to know:
- Keep a note of changes in skin integrity or possible infections.
  - o Inform the primary health care provider at the next appointment.
  - o Be sure to include information regarding skin folds.
- If there appears to be an allergy to soap, be sure to let the health care provider know this also.

National Institutes of Health. (2010). *Caregiver Guide: Tips for Caregivers of People with Alzheimer's Disease.* (NIH Publication No. 01-4013). Washington, DC: U. S. Government Printing Office.

Robinson, A., White, L., Spencer, B. (2007) *Understanding Difficult Behaviors.* Ypsilanti, Michigan: Eastern Michigan University.

Chapter 2

THE TOPIC . . . . BLADDER

The Reason for the Topic:

- Incontinence.
- Nocturia (the need to urinate frequently during the night).
- Urine odor.
- Embarrassment due to wet clothing.
- Prostate issues.
- Potential skin breakdown.
- Urinary tract infections.

Just a thought:

Imagine a woman having an embarrassing moment at an inopportune time. Unable to fly to the bathroom in time, she thinks to herself, "Does anyone know? Am I the only one that can't control my bladder?"

Actually, her dilemma happens more frequently than it should. The fear of admitting incontinence, can delay people from seeking help. Unfortunately, the longer a person waits, the more difficult it may be to treat.

Just like going to the bathroom, don't hold it. Find out what's causing the problem so you can take back control of your bladder. The treatment could easily be less complicated than the hassle of bladder problems.

Goals:

- Bladder control.
- Sleeping through the night without having to go to the bathroom.
- Intact, clear, clean skin.
- No urine odor.
- No soiled clothing or bedding.
- No bladder infections.

Interventions:

- Scheduled toileting may be helpful.
  - Don't wait until there is a need to urinate.
  - Set a timer and empty the bladder at that time even if there is no urge to void.
  - Wait one hour. (If that's too long, start at forty-five minutes.) Then empty the bladder at that time even if it there is no need to urinate.
  - Continue this process during waking hours.
  - Be sure not to skip a designated time just because it doesn't feel necessary to go to the bathroom.
  - After a few days, increase the amount of time between urinating by fifteen minutes. If there is an urgency to empty the bladder before the designated time, then do so, and re-set the timer from that point.
  - After accomplishing bladder control with that time interval for several days, then increase the time between voiding by an additional fifteen minutes.
  - Gradually increase the time between voiding until waiting for at least two hours is accomplished.

- Try to limit the intake of fluids after six pm to decrease the number of times needed to get up during the night.
  - However, don't decrease the total amount of fluid consumed during the day.
  - The body, kidneys, and bladder need fluids to function normally.
  - Daily intake of fluids needs to be at least six glasses of water per day, unless the health care provider has given directions to restrict fluids for a medical reason.
- If one of the prescribed medications is a diuretic (water pill) be sure to take it before noon.
  - This allows time for the effectiveness of the medication to rid the body of excess fluid without needing to urinate during the night.
- Try using Kegel exercises.
  - This is done by tightening the muscles used to stop urination then releasing the muscles.
    - Tighten and relax the muscles repeatedly.
  - Do this ten to twenty times at three different times during the day.
  - Do not do Kegel exercises while urinating.
    - Deliberately stopping urine when the brain is sending the message to the bladder to release urine, sends the wrong message to your brain.

Possible outcomes:
- A negative outcome is increased incontinence including the following consequences:
  - Urine odor.
  - Additional laundry.
  - Sleep disruptions.
  - Potential skin problems.

- **Positive outcomes could include:**
  - o **Bladder control.**
  - o **Improved restful sleep.**
  - o **Dry linens and clothing.**
  - o **Clean dry skin.**
  - o **No urine odor.**
- **Better understanding of prostate and bladder infections.**

When to Call for Assistance:

- **By addressing incontinence issues early a person is more likely to have successful outcomes compared to waiting until complete incontinence occurs prior to seeking help.**
- **Consider requesting a referral to an incontinence specialist.**

What the Doctor needs to know:

- **Prostate signs and symptoms are common for elderly men.**
  - o **Signs of an enlarged prostate could include:**
    - ▪ **Urinating frequently in small amounts.**
    - ▪ **Sensing the need to empty the bladder, but then having difficulty initiating the urine to flow.**
  - o **Anyone with these symptoms needs to discuss this with the primary health care provider.**
- **The symptoms of bladder infections are different in an older person compared to someone younger.**
  - o **They may not have a fever or demonstrate discomfort directly related to emptying their bladder.**
  - o **Changes in cognition, behavior, sleep, and appetite need to be reported to the primary health care provider to determine whether it would be appropriate to test for a bladder infection.**
  - o **Please note that concentrated urine does not indicate an infection.**

- It does mean that an increasing fluid intake is indicated.
  - o The presence of bacteria in urine does not always indicate that there is an infection.
- Over use of antibiotics may make it difficult to successfully treat bladder infections.

National Institute on Aging. (2013). *Age Page: Urinary Incontinence.* Washington, DC: U. S. Government Printing Office.

National Institutes of Health. (2010). *Caregiver Guide: Tips for Caregivers of People with Alzheimer's Disease.* (NIH Publication No. 01-4013). Washington, DC: U. S. Government Printing Office.

Parker, W. H., Parker, R., Rosenman, A. E. (2002). *The Incontinence Solution: Answers for Women for All Ages.* New York: Simon & Shuster.

Robinson, A., White, L., Spencer, B. (2007) *Understanding Difficult Behaviors.* Ypsilanti, Michigan: Eastern Michigan University.

Chapter 3

THE TOPIC . . . . DRIVING

The Reason for the Topic:

- **Driving is a source of independence and pride for many people.**
- **Accepting that the time may have come to stop driving can be a decision that involves a person's dignity.**
- **For individuals who lack insight regarding their cognitive decline, the topic of driving can be difficult for them to accept.**

Just a thought:

The topic of driving was discussed repeatedly at the Geriatric Assessment Clinic. The real topic wasn't driving, it was when to stop.

We knew some individuals who got lost while driving. Due to short term memory loss, no one will ever know how traumatic that was for the driver. The family clearly stated their fright of not knowing whether their loved one was safe. Imagine not knowing whether or not they would ever see them again.

So, how to approach someone who perhaps should stop driving? Respectfully. Everyone is an individual. Talking with others who know the person, the physician, and the person themselves is a place to start. Listening and empathizing need to be included.

When the decision is made, safety of other drivers must be considered. The respect and safety for passengers needs to be part of the discussion, also.

Goals:

- **Avoid preventable automobile accidents.**
- **Respect the individual while addressing a sensitive issue.**
- **Prevent a crisis.**

Interventions:

- **If there is a question whether a person can drive safely, ride with them.**
  - o **Observe for unsafe driving techniques.**
  - o **Be sure to intervene if hazardous decisions are demonstrated.**
- **Another option is to drive behind a loved one to help observe if there are concerns about their driving skills.**
- **Consider initiating a professional driving evaluation via the Department of Motor Vehicles or a local rehabilitation center.**
- **There might be a charge for an evaluation, but there is an extremely high cost if an actual accident occurs that may include injuries or even loss of life.**
  - o **The expense of testing is worth the investment in assessing driving skills.**
- **If someone gets confused where they are, they may need to have someone in the vehicle who can provide directions.**
- **Check to see if there are local driver training classes available for senior citizens.**
- **Be sure that drivers over sixty years old have their vision checked routinely for glaucoma, cataracts, and macular degeneration in addition to visual acuity.**
  - o **Refer to Chapter 20 regarding vision issues.**

Possible outcomes:

- People who were allowed to drive when they were no longer safe to do so, have caused hazardous situations including the following:
  - o Driving the wrong way on the freeway.
  - o A driver was lost for several days.
  - o Tickets even though they could not be held responsible for their actions.
  - o Accidents that were clearly preventable.
  - o Accidents with life threatening or disabling results.
- Positive outcomes include:
  - o No avoidable accidents.
  - o No driving tickets due to cognitive deficits.
  - o A respectable conclusion to a driving career.

When to Call for Assistance:

- When a person is demonstrating confusion or acts like they don't recognize their surroundings they could get lost while driving. Consider requesting cognitive testing.
- When a number of "dings" are seen on the side of a car and the person has no idea how they happened.
  - o The dents could be caused by impaired visuospatial judgment.
  - o This indicates the need to have vision and cognition testing.
- The driver has difficulty driving in or out of the garage without hitting a door.
  - o Impaired depth perception.
  - o Impaired visual acuity.
  - o Impaired visual fields.
- Driving privileges need to be discussed and possibly terminated if a person has any of the following challenges:

- o **Difficulty physically moving their legs.**
- o **Cannot turn their head forty-five degrees side to side.**
- o **If the person is taking medications for pain that could cause drowsiness.**
- **A family member can submit a request to the Department of Motor Vehicles for a driving evaluation**
  - o **This would initiate a process to evaluate a driver's ability to continue to drive safely.**

What the Doctor needs to know:

- **If a family member is apprehensive about approaching a loved one about their ability to drive, ask their health care provider to make a referral for a formal driving evaluation or neuropsychological testing.**
  - o **Due to privacy laws, a health care provider may not be allowed to discuss their patient's information with anyone unless there is consent from the patient.**
    - **Information can be provided to the health care provider from the family.**
    - **Documenting concerns and sending it to the health care provider may be helpful.**

Beerman, S., Rapport-Musson, J. (2002). *Eldercare 911*. Amherst, N.Y.: Prometheus Books.

National Institute on Aging. (2011). *Age Page: Older Drivers*. Washington, DC: U. S. Government Printing Office.

National Institutes of Health. (2010). *Caregiver Guide: Tips for Caregivers of People with Alzheimer's Disease*. (NIH Publication No. 01-4013). Washington, DC: U. S. Government Printing Office.

National Institutes of Health. (2012). *Alzheimer's Disease; Fact Sheet*. (NIH Publication No. 11-6423). Washington, DC: U. S. Government Printing Office.

Chapter 4

THE TOPIC . . . . FALLS

The Reason for the Topic:

- **Many elderly people fall and fracture a hip.**
- **Subsequently, they may lose their independence.**
- **Many falls are preventable.**

Just a thought:

Participating in the local Parkinson's Disease Support Group was enlightening for many reasons. Getting to know the individuals was a real treat. Meeting them and learning what their individual stories were taught me more about Parkinson's Disease than any text book.

Frequently, the topic of falls needed to be addressed. Then someone suggested a related concern. Learning how to get up off the floor after falling was an equal apprehension. However, there was an additional issue related to the discussion of falls.

What if the caregiver is injured as a result of assisting someone after they have fallen? Preventing falls is the best solution to this set of problems. Knowing what to do when a person falls is vital to the safety of both the one who fell and their caregiver.

Goals:

- **No falls.**
- **Be aware of potential times and locations where falls might likely occur.**

Interventions:

- **Be aware that blood pressure may drop when rising from a seated position. This is called orthostasis.**
  - o **Have blood pressure monitored when sitting, then stand and recheck the blood pressure.**
  - o **If the systolic pressure (the top number) drops by more than twenty points, the person is at risk for falling when they stand up from a seated position.**
- **Be aware of loose rugs.**
  - o **If you have one foot on the rug and the other is on the floor, then turn, the rug may slip out from underneath you.**
  - o **Either remove the rug or tack it down securely.**
- **Be sure to have grab bars in the bath tub or shower.**
  - o **Falling in the bathroom is especially dangerous since items are closer than in other rooms.**
  - o **There is an increased likelihood of injuries.**
  - o **Suction cup grab bars can be placed conveniently for someone to steady themselves to prevent falling when they enter or exit the bath tub.**
  - o **Refer to Chapter 51 for additional discussion how to assure safety in the bathroom.**
- **Be sure lighting is adequate during hours when there is no daylight.**
  - o **Inability to see objects while walking may contribute to falls.**
  - o **Have a night light on when getting out of bed to avoid tripping.**
- **Be sure shoes and slippers have non-skid soles.**
- **Be sure all floors are free of spills or any wetness.**

- If someone has been instructed to use a cane or walker, be sure the assistive device is always readily available.
  - o Encourage them to use the devices.
- To prevent someone from falling out of bed, try the following:
  - o Roll a small blanket lengthwise.
  - o Place the rolled up blanket on the side of the bed where the person gets in and out of bed.
  - o It should be placed directly on top of the mattress close to the side of the bed.
  - o Allow the top of the blanket roll to flap over toward the center of the bed. (When the person is in the bed, that part of the blanket will be underneath the person).
  - o Place a fitted sheet over the blanket.
  - o If the bed is adjacent to a wall, then only one side needs to have the blanket roll.
  - o If a person can get out of either side, then place blanket rolls on both sides.
  - o When the person needs to get out of bed, reach under the sheet and allow the blanket to un-roll.
  - o This will allow the rolled part of the blanket to drop to the floor.
  - o They won't need to climb out over the top of the blanket.
  - o If there isn't a small blanket available, a large bath towel can be used.

Possible outcomes:

- The worst outcome is a lost independence due to an injury.
- The best outcome is no falls.
- The next best outcome is no injuries if there is a fall.

When to Call for Assistance:

- When someone is on the floor, be sure they are not injured prior to assisting them to sit or stand.
- A caregiver should not try to help someone up from the floor if they could also be injured. Call 911 for assistance.
  - o Emergency personnel are trained to assess whether the person who fell may need to be taken to the emergency room.

What the Doctor Needs to Know:

- Be sure to let the primary health care provider know if you notice imbalance when rising from a seated position.
- Be sure the health care provider is aware of falls.
  - o If the cause of the fall is known, that is helpful.
- Be sure the health care provider is aware of pain that has been noticed since the fall.
- Discuss the option of having a falls assessment by a physical therapist.
  - o The physical therapist will be helpful to determine whether a cane or walker is needed to prevent falls and keep a person ambulatory.
  - o The physical therapist may have suggestions to maintain strength and mobility to prevent falls.

Beerman, S., Rapport-Musson, J. (2002). *Eldercare 911.* Amherst, N.Y.: Prometheus Books.

National Institute on Aging. (2012) *Age Page: Arthritis Advice.* Washington, DC: U. S. Government Printing Office.

National Institute on Aging. (2012). *Age Page: Falls and Fractures.* Washington, DC: U. S. Government Printing Office.

National Institute on Aging. (2014) *Age Page: Exercise and Physical Activity: Getting Fit for Life.* Washington, DC: U. S. Government Printing Office.

National Institutes of Health. (2010). *Caregiver Guide: Tips for Caregivers of People with Alzheimer's Disease.* (NIH Publication No. 01-4013). Washington, DC: U. S. Government Printing Office.

National Institutes of Health. (2013). *Age Page: Osteoporosis: The Bone Thief.* Washington, DC: U. S. Government Printing Office.

Parkinson's Disease. (2012). In NIH online publication: *Senior Health.* Retrieved from: http://nihseniorhealth.gov/parkinsonsdisease/whatisparkinsonsdisease/01.html.

Chapter 5

THE TOPIC . . . . FEET

The Reason for the Topic:

- **Continue to be ambulatory.**
- **Healthy feet are essential for a quality lifestyle**.

Just a thought:

Probably one part of the body that is ignored way too often is the foot. More accurately, feet. We stand on them. Complain when they ache. Assume they will help us travel everywhere we need to go.

Sometimes, even when they start telling us there is a problem, we continue to think about other concerns in our day. Then comes the moment when due to an infection or an injury our feet won't stand for one more minute . . . then what?

Here is an idea. How about giving feet the attention they deserve before a problem steps forward.

Goals:

- **Routine nail care with observation for wounds or infections.**
- **No open wounds.**
- **Pain free feet.**

Interventions:

- Routine foot care is essential for diabetics. A person trained in diabetic nail care is optimal for toenail trimming.

- Observe for cracks between the toes and on the bottom of the foot while trimming toenails.

- After any bathing or foot soaking be sure to dry off the foot very thoroughly especially between the toes.

Possible outcomes:

- Worst outcome is loss of feet.

- Best outcome is dry, clean feet, toes, and nails.

When to Call for Assistance:

- If a person is diabetic, any changes in the color or temperature of the feet or toes need to be addressed immediately.

What the Doctor Needs to Know:

- Be sure to report all concerns about pain, cracks that won't heal, or open areas on the feet to the primary health care provider.

National Institutes of Health. (2010). *Caregiver Guide: Tips for Caregivers of People with Alzheimer's Disease.* (NIH Publication No. 01-4013). Washington, DC: U. S. Government Printing Office.

Chapter 6

THE TOPIC . . . . HEARING/EARS

The Reason for the Topic:

- **Communication.**
- **Not missing out on topics of discussion.**
- **Being able to socialize.**
- **Being able to enjoy sounds like birds, music, nature, etc.**

Just a thought:

When a person's ability to hear is challenged, processing verbal information can take longer. If a second topic of discussion is initiated, the person with hearing loss may miss that subject. Later, when the latter topic is mentioned, the person with hearing loss may claim they knew nothing about it. There appears to be a memory loss. Actually, it is a hearing problem.

When I mentioned this scenario to patients and their families at the Geriatric Assessment Clinic, usually they all nodded in agreement without any discussion.

Goals:

- Be able to communicate fluently.
- Not to appear to have a memory problem unless there is a cognitive decline.
- Be able to hear and enjoy sounds.

Interventions:

- First, be sure there is no accumulation of earwax.
  - o There are over the counter ear cleaning products that are safe for removing ear wax.
- Don't poke any item in the ear. This includes cotton swabs.
- If a person demonstrates a delay in responding, it is advisable to have their hearing evaluated by an audiologist.
- If someone uses hearing aids for the first time, they need time to adjust to a number of factors.
  - o The following is list of adjustments to wearing hearing aids.
    - The pressure of the presence of the device itself. Usually, with time this pressure is no longer noticeable.
    - The sudden awareness of all the noises in an environment.
    - People may not realize all the little sounds around them.
    - The brain needs time to adjust to all the sounds so it can sort out the sounds it chooses to focus on hearing.
  - o The loss of quietness of the hearing impaired world needs to be respected.
    - Please realize that sometimes people with hearing impairment grieve the loss of their quiet world when they first use hearing aids.
    - In order to adjust to the change from quiet to a world of sound, they need time to accept the difference.

- **Routine checkups to assure hearing aids are functioning well may be helpful.**
  - o **The person may continue to have declining hearing and not realize it.**
  - o **The hearing aids may need to be adjusted periodically.**

Possible outcomes:
- **Negative outcomes include:**
  - o **The determination that there is a cognitive loss with no effort to correct the hearing deficit.**
  - o **Loss of socialization resulting in a reduced quality of life.**
  - o **Unable to participate in activities that were once meaningful, e.g. singing, listening to music, hearing birds sing, etc.**
- **The best outcomes include:**
  - o **More alert interactions with others.**
  - o **Participation in more social events.**
  - o **Conversing more readily with others.**
  - o **Less seemingly forgetful.**
  - o **Enjoying meaningful activities such as music.**

When to Call for Assistance:
- **If you notice a person needs to have the TV louder than they previously did, they need to at least have their ears checked for ear wax.**
  - o **This will help to determine if they need a hearing evaluation.**
- **If a person is asking to repeat what you have said it may be due to hearing loss.**
- **If a person demonstrates missing parts of conversations, consider determining if the cause is cognitive or a hearing issue.**

- A person may need a hearing evaluation if they repeat a word they thought they heard and it sounds similar to the first word but doesn't make sense in the context of the conversation.

  o For example, one person says, "Please pass the bread." Then the hearing impaired person questions, "Did I ask Ted?"

What the Doctor Needs to Know:

- Be sure the primary health care provider is aware of the following concerns:

  o Ear pain.

  o Ear drainage.

  o Need for aggressive ear wax removal.

- When there is a sudden loss of hearing, call 911 or go to the nearest emergency room.

- Discuss whether a hearing evaluation or cognitive testing are indicated.

Beerman, S., Rapport-Musson, J. (2002). *Eldercare 911*. Amherst, N.Y.: Prometheus Books.

National Institutes of Health. (2010). *Caregiver Guide: Tips for Caregivers of People with Alzheimer's Disease*. (NIH Publication No. 01-4013). Washington, DC: U. S. Government Printing Office.

National Institutes of Health. (2012). *Alzheimer's Disease; Fact Sheet*. (NIH Publication No. 11-6423). Washington, DC: U. S. Government Printing Office

Robinson, A., White, L., Spencer, B. (2007) *Understanding Difficult Behaviors*. Ypsilanti, Michigan: Eastern Michigan University.

Chapter 7

THE TOPIC . . . . HOW TO COMMUNICATE WITH YOUR DOCTOR

The Reason for the Topic:

- Communication is essential to establish and maintain mutual trust.

- It is very important to understand directions in order to know the reason for the instructions.

- It is also necessary to know the responsibility of both the patient and the health care provider.

- Being prepared for office visits optimizes time for both the patient and the health care provider.

Just a thought:

Let's say there is a guy named Sam. He comes in to see his doctor. The doctor says, "Sam, how can I help you today?"

"Well, I was out walking my dog and he started to get away from me. He tugged on the leash and it kind of pulled my back."

"So," the doctor attempted to clarify, "You hurt your back."

"No, I realized that I forgot to take my pills."

"Sam, are you having trouble with your memory?"

"No, just the dog. He couldn't wait to get outside, so I forgot to take my pills just that once."

"So, then, what can I do for you today?" The doctor inquired.

"Well, I realized when I was out with the dog, I was going to pick my prescriptions."

"OK, so your point is. . ."

"I couldn't get my medications because the pharmacy told me I am out of refills and need new prescriptions."

Could he have started with that . . .?

Goals:

- **Arrive at appointments prepared.**
- **Conclude the appointment with a clear understanding of the instructions and expectations.**

Interventions:

- **Always carry a list of medications.**
  - o **Be sure the list includes prescription medications from all of the health care providers.**
  - o **Include any medications that are over the counter medications, vitamins, and supplements.**
- **Have a notebook available between appointments.**
  - o **Whenever there is a topic to discuss with the health care provider, be sure to record it in the notebook.**

- Be sure to make a note about which items are urgent and which are a lower priority.
  - o If there is more than one topic, it may not be practical to discuss all concerns at one appointment.
  - o Be sure to bring the notebook to the appointment.
  - o Prioritize the items before the appointment.
  - o There may not be time to discuss all the items on the list.
- At the beginning of the appointment, be clear about what the concerns are and how many items there are to discuss.
  - o The health care provider may need to help prioritize which issues need to be postponed for a subsequent appointment.
- Take notes during the appointment.
- When the health care provider gives instructions, repeat the instructions back so they can be sure the instructions are understood.
  - o This will allow explanation for how important it is to follow directions.
  - o It is also helpful to clarify consequences of not following the instructions as specifically ordered.
- Also, when a person sees their doctor in a public place remember he or she does not have your chart with them.
  - o The health care provider needs to not talk about your health in public to protect your privacy.

Possible outcomes:
- If an antibiotic is ordered and not taken correctly, the infection may not be adequately treated and cause further avoidable illness.
- Sometimes antidepressants take a number of weeks before any effectiveness is seen.
  - o If the effectiveness is anticipated immediately, people may stop taking a medication without giving it an adequate trial period.

- It is helpful to be aware of potential side effects so you know what to do in case those symptoms occur.

- If someone has diabetes and doesn't realize the potential risks they are taking, avoidable serious consequences could jeopardize their health and well being.

- There are many medical conditions that require life style changes, or nutritional adjustments.
  - o It is very important to know when fluids need to be increased or restricted.
  - o Salt may need to be restricted or added depending on a person's medical conditions or treatments.
  - o Other dietary restrictions could include:
    - Green leafy vegetables for patients taking Coumadin.
    - Protein intake could affect medication interactions.
  - o Be aware of all dietary and life style changes that the health care provider instructs.
    - Be sure to ask questions and clarify any concerns as necessary to be sure the instructions are clear.

When to Call for Assistance:

- When starting a new medication, if for any reason the person decides to stop taking it, be sure to let the health care provider know.
  - o There may be alternate options.
  - o There may be serious problems by not following your health care provider's instructions.

- Always call 911 if someone is having trouble breathing or becomes unconscious.

- Call 911 or go to the nearest emergency room if there is sudden swelling in the face or throat.

What the Doctor Needs to Know:

- Contact the primary health care provider if experiencing nausea, vomiting, weight loss, or fever.

- If there are mild possible side effects, write down those symptoms in the notebook to take it to the next appointment.

- When a new medication is initiated, but sure to know what the expectations are.
    - o Be aware of potential side effects.

- Before starting a new medications be sure to know if it needs to be taken at a time that correlates with food:
    - o On an empty stomach.
    - o After meals.
    - o With or without certain foods.
    - o What time it is to be taken.

- Due to privacy laws, a health care provider may not be allowed to discuss their patient's information with anyone unless there is consent from the patient.
    - ▪ Information can be provided to the health care provider from the family.
    - ▪ Documenting concerns and sending it to the health care provider may be helpful.

Beerman, S., Rapport-Musson, J. (2002). *Eldercare 911*. Amherst, N.Y.: Prometheus Books.

National Institute on Aging. (2014) *Talking with Your Doctor: A Guide for Older People*. (NIH Publication No. 05-3452). Washington, DC: U.S. Government Printing Office.

National Institutes of Health. (2010). *Caregiver Guide: Tips for Caregivers of People with Alzheimer's Disease*. (NIH Publication No. 01-4013). Washington, DC: U. S. Government Printing Office.

National Institutes of Health. (2012). *Alzheimer's Disease; Fact Sheet*. (NIH Publication No. 11-6423). Washington, DC: U. S. Government Printing Office.

Chapter 8

THE TOPIC . . . . LAUNDRY

The Reason for the Topic:

- **Having clean sheets and personal clothing promote a healthy environment.**

- **When it takes too much effort to perform laundry tasks independently, for some elderly people it simply stops happening.**

Just a thought:

One of my duties as the nurse for the Geriatric Assessment Clinic was performing home visits with patients prior to their appointment with the rest of the team. One of the concerns I always addressed was the issue of laundry.

Some people had their facilities in the basement. Then stairs became an additional issue. Others had their washing machine in one of the main rooms. However, due to a number of reasons they couldn't consistently take care of their soiled clothing, so potential falls were a concern as people tried not to trip over dirty laundry.

Then there were others who had simply stopped washing their clothes. The task had become too overwhelming due to pain, lack of physical stamina, memory, or a number of issues common to aging.

Sometimes seeking help indicates a loss of independence. So laundry that no longer can be accomplished the way it once did, has translated into a safety issue.

Goals:

- Be sure laundry facilities are available with safe access.

- People who are no longer able to perform this task due to declining dexterity and strength have assistance with changing bed linens.

- If laundry facilities are in the basement assure safe transit of laundry items to prevent falls.

Interventions:

- Participating in folding clean clothes may be rewarding for people. Encourage an individual to do as much for themselves as possible.

- If a person is reluctant to change clothing, then make sure clean clothes are in sight and readily available.

    o Refer to Problem Behaviors Chapter 35.

- If standing becomes an issue due to fatigue, be sure there is a chair available in the laundry room to sit on as needed.

- If arrangements can be made to have the washer and dryer on the main floor, this will provide convenience and safety.

- If the only place to do laundry is down a flight of stairs take extra caution.

    o Be sure hand railings are sturdy.

    o Be sure lighting is adequate.

    o Encourage people to allow items to drop to the basement floor so that they don't need to carry items in their hands down the stairs.

        ▪ It may be too difficult to carry laundry and see the stairs simultaneously, increasing the chance of falling.

        ▪ Consider employing someone to help with laundry if a person is unsafe going to the basement and does not realize the potential danger.

        ▪ Consider locking the door to the basement to prohibit avoidable accidents.

Possible outcomes:

- Negative outcomes could include:
  - o Laundry not done.
  - o Illness as a result of unhealthy living environment.
  - o Injuries due to falling down the stairs.
- Positive outcomes may include:
  - o Clean linens routinely.
  - o No injuries from performing laundry tasks.
  - o A sense of accomplishment from participating in a lifelong task.

When to Call for Assistance:

- If a person isn't aware of potential safety hazards related to laundry, consider having someone assess the situation for safety.
  - o This can provide an unbiased opinion.
  - o Some people would prefer to hear suggestions from someone other than a family member.

What the Doctor Needs to Know:

- The physician only needs to be involved if a health issue results from the concerns discussed previously in this chapter.

National Institutes of Health. (2012). *Alzheimer's Disease; Fact Sheet.* (NIH Publication No. 11-6423). Washington, DC: U. S. Government Printing Office.

Beerman, S., Rapport-Musson, J. (2002). *Eldercare 911.* Amherst, N.Y.: Prometheus Books.

National Institute on Aging. (2012). *There's No Place Like Home – For Growing Old: Tips from the National Institute on Aging.* Washington, DC: U. S. Government Printing Office.

National Institute on Aging. (2007). *So Far Away: Twenty Questions for Long-distance Caregivers.* (NIH Publication No: 05-5496). Washington, DC: U. S. Government Printing Office.

National Institutes of Health. (2010). *Caregiver Guide: Tips for Caregivers of People with Alzheimer's Disease.* (NIH Publication No. 01-4013). Washington, DC: U. S. Government Printing Office.

Chapter 9

THE TOPIC . . . . LIVING ALONE & HOW TO CALL FOR HELP

The Reason for the Topic:

- One way to maintain independence at home is to have a way to call for help in case of an emergency.
- If a person fell in the bathroom, how close is the nearest phone?
  - o Would they be able to reach it?
- Individuals who have basements or rooms upstairs have a higher risk for falling and injuries.

Just a thought:

One of worst accidents a person could have is slipping in the bath tub and not being able to get up. I have watched the eyes of many people as I explained the stories of individuals who have fallen and not been found until the next day.

I have conferred with individuals who feel that to have a call system is unnecessary. But as I discuss detail by detail what the night would be like for them if they fell at 11:00 pm and were not found for twelve long hours. Those endless hours of helpless loneliness could be avoided by having an emergency call system.

Some people feel that to have a call system implies they aren't independent. The reality is that a call systems supports independence.

Goals:

- Always be able to call for help.

Interventions:

- There are a variety of call alert systems available. Local agencies may be able to assist with obtaining the device.
  - o Area Agency on Aging.
  - o Commission on Aging.
  - o Local Support Groups.
- If a person is resistant to having a call system installed, discuss the consequences of specific emergency situations.
- Sometimes elderly couples reside together.
  - o In some situations one of them may be cognitively impaired.
  - o The individual that is higher functioning needs to have a call system in case of an emergency since their partner cannot call for help.
- Be sure that the individual understands that the call system device can get wet.
  - o They should not take it off in the shower or bath tub.
- Be sure that the individual is always wearing the device twenty-four hours a day.
  - o If they take it off at night, then fall in the bathroom, they won't be able to reach the device.

Possible outcomes:

- A potential adverse outcome is if a person falls and does not remember they have a call system.
- Sometimes people have a call system, but don't keep it with them.

- o Then when an emergency happens, they can't reach the device.
- o They can't call for help if they don't have the device with them.
- The best outcome is when a person needs help and can call for help immediately wherever they are.

When to Call for Assistance:
- There are a number of choices of emergency call systems.
- Establish a system prior to a crisis.

What the Doctor Needs to Know:
- If you feel your loved one is not safe to be live alone due to declining cognition or physical reasons, discuss your concerns with their health care provider.
  - o Refer to Chapter 7.
- Having cognitive testing to determine a person's ability not only to remember but also to plan and solve problems could help to determine if they are safe to live alone.

National Institute on Aging. (2007). *So Far Away: Twenty Questions for Long-distance Caregivers.* (NIH Publication No: 05-5496). Washington, DC: U. S. Government Printing Office.

National Institutes of Health. (2010). *Caregiver Guide: Tips for Caregivers of People with Alzheimer's Disease.* (NIH Publication No. 01-4013). Washington, DC: U. S. Government Printing Office.

National Institute on Aging. (2012). *There's No Place Like Home – For Growing Old: Tips from the National Institute on Aging.* Washington, DC: U. S. Government Printing Office.

Cowley, G. (2000). Alzheimer's Disease: Unlocking the Mystery. *Newsweek.* (January).

Chapter 10

THE TOPIC . . . . MEDICATIONS

<u>The Reason for the Topic:</u>

- **Medications are ordered for a reason.**

    o **The only way to know if the medications are helpful or causing adverse side effects is to be sure that medications are taken as ordered.**

- **There may be a number of reasons why elderly patients don't take medications as prescribed.**

    o **Sometimes they can't do it.**

    o **Other times they choose not to.**

- **Health care providers need to know exactly what medications a person is taking in order to make necessary adjustments in medications or dosages.**

- **Many people choose to self-prescribe over the counter medications without notifying the provider who is responsible for prescription medications.**

    o **There may be significant drug interactions that an individual does not realize.**

Just a thought:

*There are times when I really appreciated being a nurse. There are times when I was exceptionally thankful that I am **not** a pharmacist. Many times people would bring their medication bottles with them to their Geriatric Assessment Clinic appointments. Bags of prescription bottles were carted into the room. The pharmacist would then try to sort out what the patient was actually consuming. Did I mention how much I appreciate pharmacists?*

After reviewing the mound of bottles, it never ceased to amaze me that no one knew exactly what pills were actually being taken. Many prescriptions had been filled several months previously. But there was still a significant quantity of pills in the container.

What can be learned? If someone has a complicated list of medications with multiple times to be taken per day, perhaps it would be a good idea to review how and when and if they are really taking the pills.

Goals:

- **Correct medications are taken as ordered.**
- **Simplify the number of times medications need to be taken per day.**
- **Use a weekly pill organizer.**

Interventions:

- **If medications are taken out of the prescription bottle each time a pill is to be taken, it is more difficult to track accuracy.**
- **Use a weekly pill box to be sure a person is remembering to take their medications as prescribed.**
  - o **It is not good for medications to be missed.**
  - o **It may be very dangerous if a person forgot that they had already taken their pills, then overdose by taking the next day's medications.**
- **If a person cannot safely be responsible for taking their medications accurately, then another adult needs to accept the task of ordering, setting up, and monitoring administration of medications. If the individual continues to have problems taking medications accurately,**

then someone needs to actually hand the pills to the person at the correct time and verify that the medications are swallowed.

- Always carry a list of medications including prescription drugs and over the counter medications.

- When a new medication is ordered, be sure to ask the ordering health care provider the following information:
  - o What is it for?
  - o What time of day should it be taken?
  - o Should it be taken with food or on an empty stomach?
  - o Are there certain foods to avoid while taking the new medication?
  - o What should be expected from the medication?
  - o What side effects might happen?
  - o Is there a reason the health care provider needs to be contacted? If so, what needs to be discussed?

Possible outcomes:

- The best outcome is that medications are taken as prescribed.

- A poor outcome is someone forgetting to take the medications and suffering from the lack of treatment.

- A worse outcome is when someone with Diabetes, high blood pressure, or other serious medical conditions, does not take medications as prescribed and avoidable hospital admissions occur.

- A crisis could result if medications are taken more frequently than prescribed or stopped without informing the health care provider.

- Adverse outcomes could also result when over the counter supplements are taken without knowing the potential drug interactions with prescription medications.

When to Call for Assistance:

- When a medication is received from a pharmacy, ask questions to be sure the directions are understood.

- **Be sure to know what to expect from taking the medication as well as what side effects may occur.**
- **Before choosing to self-prescribe over the counter medications, seek advice from the pharmacist regarding if it would safe or not.**

What the Doctor Needs to Know:

- **Always keep the health care provider informed of any medication changes.**
- **If there are additional specialists, it is important that they all know the complete list of prescription and over the counter medications.**
- **If there are suspected side effects from a prescription medication, do not stop taking the medication until informing the prescribing health care provider.**
  - o **They may choose to replace that medication with an alternate option or adjust the dosage to avoid the side effects.**
- **Call 911 in case a person is having difficulty breathing or has lost consciousness.**

Beerman, S., Rapport-Musson, J. (2002). *Eldercare 911*. Amherst, N.Y.: Prometheus Books.

Cowley, G. (2000). Alzheimer's Disease: Unlocking the Mystery. *Newsweek*. (January).

National Institute on Aging. (2007). *So Far Away: Twenty Questions for Long-distance Caregivers*. (NIH Publication No: 05-5496). Washington, DC: U. S. Government Printing Office.

National Institute on Aging. (2011) *Age Page: Aging and Your Eyes*. Washington, DC: U. S. Government Printing Office.

National Institute on Aging. (2012). *There's No Place Like Home – For Growing Old: Tips from the National Institute on Aging*. Washington, DC: U. S. Government Printing Office.

National Institute on Aging. (2013). *Age Page: Depression*. Washington, DC: U. S. Government Printing Office.

National Institute on Aging. (2014) *Talking with Your Doctor: A Guide for Older People*. (NIH Publication No. 05-3452). Washington, DC: U.S. Government Printing Office

National Institute on Aging. (2014). *Alzheimer's Disease Medications*. (NIH Publication No. 08-3431). Washington, DC: U. S. Government Printing Office.

National Institutes of Health. (2010). *Caregiver Guide: Tips for Caregivers of People with Alzheimer's Disease*. (NIH Publication No. 01-4013). Washington, DC: U. S. Government Printing Office.

Robinson, A., White, L., Spencer, B. (2007) *Understanding Difficult Behaviors*. Ypsilanti, Michigan: Eastern Michigan University.

Chapter 11

THE TOPIC . . . . MEMORY

The Reason for the Topic:

- **Memory loss is frequently assumed to be a sign of dementia.**

    o **It is important to realize there are many reasons for memory problems that may be treatable.**

- **If a person is diagnosed with dementia, there are treatments to slow down the progression of cognitive loss and preserve personal care skills.**

Just a thought:

When a person has short term memory loss, frequently they have the exact same conversation repeatedly in a very short amount of time. I actually found this to be a convenience at times.

At the Geriatric Assessment Clinic, many times a family member needed to speak with our physician without the patient in the room. It was my responsibility to keep that patient occupied in another room. Once I knew what their favorite topic was, I asked them to talk about it as if it were being discussed for the first time.

For example, if we had a patient very much attached to a little dog she had loved for many years, I would keep asking her to tell me about her pet. Periodically, she may get anxious about why she was there. Instead of explaining anything, I would simply ask her, "Do you have any pets?"

The story would start. She would regale the saga of when she first got her puppy. With twinkles in her eyes, she rattled on in detail about the favorite moments they had shared.

She could sound like she was telling it for the first time. . . repeatedly.

Goals:

- **Identify whether a person has memory deficits and, additionally, other cognitive declines:**
    - o **Decision making skills.**
    - o **Visual perception.**
    - o **Auditory memory.**
    - o **Visual memory.**
    - o **Language skills.**
- **Adjust a person's support and supervision to assure they are safe. Their needs are being met if they are incapable of meeting their own needs.**
- **Consider all possible treatment options pertinent to the cause of the memory loss.**

Interventions:

- **Discuss the benefit of neuropsychological testing if an individual demonstrates any of the following:**
    - o **Repeating themselves or asking the same questions repeatedly.**
    - o **If someone forgets appointments repeatedly.**
    - o **If a person has not been able to take their medications correctly.**
    - o **There is concern whether a person can drive safely.**
    - o **There is concern whether a person is capable of living alone.**
    - o **The individual has demonstrated difficulty managing their own finances.**
- **Neuropsychological testing will help to diagnose the following:**
    - o **Verbal memory loss.**

- o **Visual memory loss.**
- o **Problem solving skills.**
- o **Visual spatial perception.**
- o **Driving skills.**
- o **Other cognitive functions.**
- **If someone does have memory loss, it is not important for them to know what date it is.**
  - o **It may cause unnecessary struggles for the caregiver and the individual to force someone to recall information that does not matter.**
- **It is beneficial for someone with memory issues to receive a diagnosis in case the cause is treatable:**
  - o **Urinary tract infection.**
  - o **Thyroid problems.**
  - o **Depression.**
  - o **Sleep disorders.**
  - o **Hearing loss.**
  - o **Other medical conditions.**
  - o **Side effects of some medications.**
- **If someone is receiving medications for memory loss, do not assume that they will consistently remember to take their pills due to their memory problems.**
- **Make a list of specific examples of forgetfulness to take to the health care provider such as:**
  - o **Forgetting names.**
  - o **Misplacing items.**
  - o **Not remembering how to perform familiar tasks.**
- **Many people have no insight that they are demonstrating memory loss.**

- Approach a person with respect to their lack of insight by using non-threatening terms to encourage them to have an assessment for their memory loss.
  - o Tell them, "This may be a good time to be sure you are as well as you can be."
  - o Instead of saying, "We need to know if you have Alzheimer's Disease."
- Memory games may be helpful for a person to practice and preserve cognitive skills.
- Socializing can help a person practice cognitive functions.
  - o To socialize a person needs to be able to hear, comprehend, formalize responses, and state their thoughts in response.
  - o Without realizing it, carrying on a conversation utilizes multiple parts of the brain.
- Refer to Chapter 25 for further information also related to memory loss.

Possible outcomes:
- Medications for memory loss may not improve their current memory.
  - o However, if someone is taking a medication and is not declining, this may be an indication that the medication is effective.
  - o Stopping the medication may cause a noticeable decline.
- There are benefits to initiating treatment sooner than waiting.
  - o People may delay the need to move out of their homes by choosing to take medications for dementia.

When to Call for Assistance:
- It may be helpful to obtain educational information regarding memory loss from local agencies.
- Attending caregiver support groups can also provide practical information by sharing experiences.

o **Hearing what other families have learned through similar experiences may be beneficial.**

What the Doctor needs to Know:

- **Be sure a responsible adult attends medical appointments whenever a person with memory loss is seen by any health care professional.**

- **The individual may not recall why they at the appointment.**

    o **They cannot inform their health care provider what the concerns are.**

    o **Additionally, if they were given instructions by the provider, they may not recall what information was discussed.**

- **Request neuropsychological testing to determine the following:**

    o **Whether there is a cognitive disorder.**

    o **What the treatment options are.**

    o **What supervisory issues need consideration.**

    o **Is the person competent to make decisions.**

Beerman, S., Rapport-Musson, J. (2002). *Eldercare 911*. Amherst, N.Y.: Prometheus Books.

National Institutes of Health. (2010). *Caregiver Guide: Tips for Caregivers of People with Alzheimer's Disease.*

Caregiver Guide: Tips for Caregivers of People with Alzheimer's Disease. (NIH Publication No. 01- 4013). Washington, DC: U. S. Government Printing Office.

Cowley, G. (2000). Alzheimer's Disease: Unlocking the Mystery. *Newsweek.* (January).

Kalb, C. (2000). Coping with the Darkness: Revolutionary new approaches in providing care are helping people with Alzheimer's stay active and feel productive. *Newsweek.* (January).

National Institute on Aging. (2014). *Alzheimer's Disease Medications.* (NIH Publication No. 08-3431). Washington, DC: U. S. Government Printing Office.

National Institutes of Health. (2012). *Alzheimer's Disease; Fact Sheet.* (NIH Publication No. 11-6423). Washington, DC: U. S. Government Printing Office.

Chapter 12

THE TOPIC .... MOBILITY

The Reason for the Topic:

- **The best thing a person can do for general health is remain ambulatory for as many years possible.**

- **Walking helps to keep your bones strong.**

- **It also promotes circulation and oxygen to your muscles and brain.**

- **Mood state can also benefit from walking.**

- **Mobility helps a person remain independent.**

Just a thought:

Imagine that your eighty year old mother has a doctor's appointment on the second floor of the medical building. Your father is coming to the appointment with the two of you. To complicate matters he is in a wheel chair.

While waiting at the clinic, there is a fire drill. You are told that everyone must be evacuated, but you can't use the elevator. Perched at the top of the stairs with two disabled parents and only one of you, what do you do?

Fortunately, the drill is completed and the descent is not required. But what if there were a real fire? What is the solution to this equation?

Mobility is truly a treasure.

Goals:

- **Prevent falls and injuries.**
- **Enjoy the independence that walking provides.**
- **Stay mobile.**

Interventions:

- **Walk every day.**
- **Find a place that is easy and convenient to walk daily.**
- **People who live in apartments can walk in hallways so they do not need to walk outside when the weather is not favorable.**
- **If you watch TV or do a lot of sitting, every time there is a commercial stand up and walk around the room.**
- **Schedule walking into your daily routine.**
- **Schedule walking into your weekly routine.**
- **Schedule time to walk with someone.**
  - o **This will help to keep a walking schedule and provide time to socialize.**

Possible outcomes:

- **Better quality of life because of remaining ambulatory.**
- **Best outcome is an independent life style due to mobility.**
- **Worst outcome is lost independence due to declining mobility.**

When to Call for Assistance:

- **Sometimes it can be helpful to have assistive devices, such as a cane or walker.**

- **If using an assistive device allows you to stay mobile, then realize it is a tool for independence.**

- **It may be helpful to have an occupational therapist evaluate the home setting to suggest how the situation may be adapted to promote the highest level of mobility and safety.**

What the Doctor Needs to Know:

- **If you are concerned about the potential for falls or imbalance, ask your health care provider for a physical therapy referral.**

- **Consider requesting an occupational therapy referral:**

  - **An example could be tools to help with independent dressing.**

  - **A kitchen organization analysis may be helpful for meal preparation.**

Beerman, S., Rapport-Musson, J. (2002). *Eldercare 911.* Amherst, N.Y.: Prometheus Books.

National Institute on Aging. (2012). *Age Page: Falls and Fractures.* Washington, DC: U. S. Government Printing Office.

National Institute on Aging. (2014) *Age Page: Exercise and Physical Activity: Getting Fit for Life.* Washington, DC: U. S. Government Printing Office.

National Institutes of Health. (2010). *Caregiver Guide: Tips for Caregivers of People with Alzheimer's Disease.* (NIH Publication No. 01-4013). Washington, DC: U. S. Government Printing Office.

National Institutes of Health. (2014). *Lewy Body Dementia: Information for Patients, Families, and Professionals.* (NIH Publication 13-7907). Washington, DC: U. S. Government Printing Office.

Parkinson's Disease. (2012). In NIH online publication: *Senior Health.* Retrieved from: http://nihseniorhealth.gov/parkinsonsdisease/whatisparkinsonsdisease/01.html.

Chapter 13

THE TOPIC . . . . MONITORING FINANCES

The Reason for the Topic:

- **As people age, they may no longer be able to keep accurate track of their finances independently.**
    - o **This can lead to missed bill payments.**
    - o **If bills are not paid, utility services may be shut off.**
- **Elderly people have frequently been the victims of scams and lost significant amounts of money.**

Just a thought:

During my years at the Geriatric Assessment Clinic, unfortunately, we witnessed many individuals being taken advantage of financially. It was sad to listen to family members tell their stories of suddenly finding out their money was gone.

Financial crises included everything from having their electricity shut off due to forgetting to pay bills all the way to "contributing" to scams over the phone. This presents only samples of situations where elderly people needed guidance to protect their assets and assure monthly payments were completed when they were due.

Making proactive arrangements are much more cost effective than trying to sort out an avoidable crisis later.

Goals:

- All bills are paid on time.
- No funds are lost due to scams or an inability to manage finances.
- Plans are established for Durable Power of Attorney (DPOA) documents prior to a crisis.
  - o This includes financial and medical advocacy.

Interventions:

- If a person is receiving mail that are potential scams, consider having mail forwarded to an adult child.
  - o Request junk mail to be stopped.
- Be sure that financial accounts are being monitored by a responsible adult.
- Most financial institutions have systems in place to monitor for potential fraud.
  - o Discuss this with your bank or credit union to find out their policies and procedures for protecting funds.

Possible outcomes:

- Best outcome includes finances are handled proactively and there are no crises.
- Worst case scenario is personal funds lost due to fraud or financial abuse.

When to Call for Assistance:

- It is advisable to seek legal assistance for establishing a Durable Power of Attorney for finances and medical decision making.
- Many health institutions have forms and guidance for establishing end of life wishes as well as patient advocacy.
- If fraud or abuse is suspected, be sure to notify the appropriate agency to investigate.
- Consider contacting protective services to help assess the situation.

<u>What the Doctor Needs to Know:</u>

- **If a person has become incompetent to make decisions for themselves, documents usually need at least one physician, and frequently two, to dictate a statement of incompetency for the advocate to be allowed to make decisions for that individual.**

- **To establish whether a person is competent to make legal decision, neuropsychological testing may be indicated.**

Beerman, S., Rapport-Musson, J. (2002). *Eldercare 911*. Amherst, N.Y.: Prometheus Books.

National Institute on Aging. (2012). *Age Page: Getting Your Affairs in Order*. Washington, DC: U. S. Government Printing Office.

National Institute on Aging. (2013). *Legal and Financial Planning for People with Alzheimer's Disease*. (NIH Publication No. 08-6422). Washington, DC: U.S. Government Printing Office.

National Institute on Aging. (2014) *Advance Care Planning: Tips from the National Institute on Aging.*

National Institutes of Health. (2010). *Caregiver Guide: Tips for Caregivers of People with Alzheimer's Disease*. (NIH Publication No. 01-4013). Washington, DC: U. S. Government Printing Office.

National Institutes of Health. (2012). *Alzheimer's Disease; Fact Sheet*. (NIH Publication No. 11-6423). Washington, DC: U. S. Government Printing Office.

Chapter 14

THE TOPIC . . . . NUTRITION

The Reason for the Topic:

- Balanced nutrition is vital at any age, but nourishment for elderly people is a basic essential for healthy living.

- Many disease processes are affected by nutrition.

- Certain medications need to be given in direct association with food:

    o On an empty stomach.

    o After meals.

    o Avoid certain specific types of foods.

- These instructions may not be easy for elderly people to remember.

- Poor nutrition can complicate many disease processes.

- When a person becomes forgetful, they may not remember to eat routinely.

- Limited incomes sometimes contribute to poor nutritional choices.

Just a thought:

The stories I could relay about the contents of people's kitchens could fill more pages than you could imagine. People who could tell me how they followed their diabetic diet would have donuts and cookies piled on the counter. Others would tell me how much they enjoyed getting prepared meals. But then why was the freezer filled with those meals?

I think the kitchens that concerned me the most were the ones that were absolutely spotless. Nothing was there. No messy sink or dirty stove. In fact, there was not any food to be found either.

So, did they go out to eat for every meal. Were they eating . . . anything?

Goals:

- **Appropriate caloric intake for an individual's current weight.**
- **Adjustment in caloric intake based on an individual's desired weight.**
- **Balanced nutrition.**
- **Dietary guidelines are followed as indicated by medication interactions and medical necessity.**
    - o **Know which medications are to be taken with food.**
    - o **Know which medications need to be taken on an empty stomach.**
    - o **Follow the guidelines for Coumadin regarding green vegetable intake.**
    - o **Be sure fluid intake correlates with treatment for heart failure, kidney failure, etc.**
- **Appropriate type carbohydrate intake for Diabetics.**
    - o **Understanding the difference between complex carbohydrates and simple carbohydrates.**
        - ▪ **Vegetables and fruits vs. sugary foods.**
- **When a person has a medical diagnosis be sure that all dietary restrictions and guidelines are understood and followed.**

Interventions:

- Observe what foods are readily available in the kitchen.
- For people who eat out frequently:
  - Where do they usually go?
  - What types of food do they tend to order?
- For individuals who have been losing weight or not consuming an adequate balanced intake, consider adding a supplement.
  - This could be a readymade supplement or a powdered breakfast drink.
  - There are many options available at local pharmacies.
  - Be sure that added supplements are provided between meals. The supplements can be very filling.
  - If the person chooses to drink the supplement, they may be too full to eat the meal.
  - All that is accomplished in that situation is trading calories and not adding nutritional benefit.
  - Provide meal supplements and snacks two hours before or after meals.
- Be sure that fiber and fluid intake are adequate to promote a normal bowel pattern.
- Constipation is a frequent struggle due to the aging process and some types of medications.
  - Adding fruit such as prunes or apples may help to regulate bowels.

Possible outcomes:

- Best outcomes are:
  - Stable weight in a healthy range.
  - Effective medications taken at the correct times in correlation with food intake.

- o Stable blood sugar control.
- o Stable laboratory values indicating adequate protein levels, and pertinent findings the health care provider is monitoring.
- o Laboratory studies show correct dietary intake of foods with specified limitations, e.g. levels monitored to manage Coumadin indicate consistent intake of green vegetables.

- Worst outcomes are:
  - o Unwanted weight loss.
  - o Prolonged illness due to inadequate protein intake.
  - o Blood sugars out of control.
  - o Non-steady blood thinning levels for people taking Coumadin.
  - o Ineffective medications because of not being taken on an empty stomach.
  - o Fluid retention.

When to Call for Assistance:

- When a patient is given a medical diagnosis that could be affected by their dietary intact, consider requesting a referral to a dietician.
  - o This could assist to develope a daily food guideline.
  - o This could help someone to understand the consequences of not following a dietary plan.

What the Doctor Needs to Know:

- Discuss the following issues with the primary health care provider:
  - o If weight loss is a concern, is there a medical cause?
  - o Would any diagnostic tests be indicated?
  - o Be sure to clarify if alcohol is medically contraindicated for the patient's diagnosis.
  - o Are their potential adverse drug interactions if alcohol is consumed with the patient's medications?

- Are their specific dietary or fluid limitations?

- If the person's weights have been recorded, be sure to bring the list of weights to appointments with health care providers.

- If constipation has become problematic, discuss options with the health care provider.

National Institutes of Health. (2013). *What's on Your Plate: Smart Food Choices for Healthy Aging.* (Publication No. 11-7708). Washington, DC: U. S. Government Printing Office.

Robinson, A., White, L., Spencer, B. (2007) *Understanding Difficult Behaviors.* Ypsilanti, Michigan: Eastern Michigan University.

National Institutes of Health. (2010). *Caregiver Guide: Tips for Caregivers of People with Alzheimer's Disease.* (NIH Publication No. 01-4013). Washington, DC: U. S. Government Printing Office.

Beerman, S., Rapport-Musson, J. (2002). *Eldercare 911.* Amherst, N.Y.: Prometheus Books.

Chapter 15

THE TOPIC . . . . PAIN

The Reason for the Topic:

- **Pain is a subjective issue.**
- **For elderly patients, pain can cause other issues:**
    - o **Limited self care.**
    - o **Decreased sleep.**
    - o **Inadequate nutrition.**
    - o **Compromised independence.**

Just a thought:

Pain is a subjective complaint. However, when a person has advanced dementia, they may not be able to accurately convey their comfort needs.

Many times I witnessed individuals who were asked if they were in pain, would smile and say, "No, I'm fine." But then no less than two minutes later, they would wince in distress as they attempted to walk.

Others were seen crying at night, only to tell someone the next day what a pleasant night's sleep they enjoyed. The objective of assessing pain, needs to be much more than subjective.

Goals:

- Daily pain control.

- No inadvertent over-dosing of pain medication.

Interventions:

- Be sure that the health care provider knows all the pain issues.

- When asked directly, an elderly patient may readily minimize their pain and say, "I'm fine." This may not be accurate information.

- Dementia patients frequently can grimace and cry in pain for hours, then when asked, deny they are having any pain.

- When someone has short term memory loss, they may not be able to convey their pain complaints.

- Document a complete description of pain when it is objectively observed:

  o Where is the pain?

  o What type of pain? (sharp/dull/radiating/piercing)

  o When does it hurt?

  o When did it start?

  o How long does the pain last?

  o What treatments have been tried?

- Consider having a discussion with the health care provider whether a referral for physical therapy or other diagnostic services could be helpful.

- Try using non-medication treatments:

  o Make in ice pack that can be pliable.

    ▪ Use a quart size plastic zip-lock bag.

    ▪ Pour one cup water and one half cup rubbing alcohol into the zip-lock bag.

    ▪ Freeze for at least one hour.

    ▪ The ice bag will mold to a body part.

  o After the ice has melted, re-freeze the bag of fluid.

- **Consider using heat.**
    - o **Never use high heat.**
    - o **Moist heat can be applied using a wet wash cloth to the painful area.**
    - o **Then place a water proof covering over the heating pad.**
    - o **Never use heat for more than ten to fifteen minutes at a time.**
    - o **Observe the skin after every time a heating pad is used.**
    - o **Be aware of redness and potential burns.**
    - o **Remember elderly people tend to have sensitive skin.**
- **Pillows may provide support.**
    - o **Try different sizes.**
    - o **Some pillows provide softer cushion than others.**
    - o **Small blankets may provide adaptable support for an arm or a leg.**
- **Encourage a person to find a position of comfort.**
    - o **Most people need to be repositioned routinely.**
- **If an individual is not capable of following instructions, then a responsible adult needs to provide supervision and assistance to aid in pain management.**
- **Try to determine precipitating factors.**
    - o **What is causing the pain or discomfort?**
    - o **Do the treatments make the pain worse?**

Possible outcomes:
- **Positive outcome is adequate/improved pain control.**
- **Poor outcome is no change in pain control.**
- **The worst outcome is a crisis as the result of not following instructions for pain management.**

When to Call for Assistance:

- **After receiving an assessment of the pain, be sure to let the health care provider know if the treatment is not being followed for whatever reason.**

- **After receiving an assessment of the pain, be sure to let the health care provider know if the treatment is inadequate.**

What the Doctor Needs to Know:

- **Be sure the health care provider has all the information describing the pain.**

    o **Be sure objective documentation is included.**

- **If the prescribed treatment does not help or if the change in treatment makes the pain worse, be sure to let the health care provider know.**

Beerman, S., Rapport-Musson, J. (2002). *Eldercare 911.* Amherst, N.Y.: Prometheus Books.

National Institute on Aging. (2012) *Age Page: Arthritis Advice.* Washington, DC: U. S. Government Printing Office.

National Institute on Aging. (2012). *Age Page: Falls and Fractures.* Washington, DC: U. S. Government Printing Office

National Institute on Aging. (2014) *Age Page: Exercise and Physical Activity: Getting Fit for Life.* Washington, DC: U. S. Government Printing Office.

National Institute on Aging. (2014). *Alzheimer's Disease Medications.* (NIH Publication No. 08-3431). Washington, DC: U. S. Government Printing Office.

National Institutes of Health. (2010). *Caregiver Guide: Tips for Caregivers of People with Alzheimer's Disease.* (NIH Publication No. 01-4013). Washington, DC: U. S. Government Printing Office.

National Institutes of Health. (2012). *Alzheimer's Disease; Fact Sheet.* (NIH Publication No. 11-6423). Washington, DC: U. S. Government Printing Office.

U. S. Department of Health and Human Services, National Institutes of Health. (2013). *Your Guide to Healthy Sleep.* (NIH Publication No. 11-5271.6) Washington, DC: U.S. Government Printing Office.

Chapter 16

THE TOPIC .... PERSONAL CARE

The Reason for the Topic:

- Sometimes as people age, taking care of themselves becomes a struggle due to number of issues:
    - o Pain.
    - o Limited range of arm reach.
    - o Declining visual acuity.
    - o Declining mobility.
- Due to the prevalence of depression in the elderly, sometimes a person might lose interest in their own personal care.
- Slowness is a typical part of the aging process.
    - o Younger family members need to realize and accept that more time needs to be allowed for an individual to care for themselves.
    - o This may mean, an older person might need to be reminded to start preparing earlier for whatever event is planned.

Just a thought:

During a session at a Parkinson's Disease support group meeting, people were discussing their personal stories. Several people said they had begun to lose their balance and had fallen a few times. Others had noticed a tremor that they couldn't stop. Slowness can be a one of the primary symptoms, also.

Repeatedly, people would discuss how they had to allow extra time to get out the door to get to appointments on time. Mornings translated into a series of time consuming tasks that previously hadn't required even a thought to accomplish.

Nevertheless, independence, no matter how much effort or time, was always worth the endeavor.

Goals:

- **Maintain independence as many years as a person is physically able.**
- **Support an individual's dignity, privacy, and respect.**
- **Prioritize details for the individual as long as safety is not an issue.**

Interventions:

- **Observe the individual for lapses in personal care:**
    - o **Unkempt appearance.**
    - o **Poor nail care.**
    - o **Soiled clothing.**
    - o **Body odor.**
- **Discuss your concerns with the person.**
    - o **They may not have realized the changes you have witnessed.**
    - o **When discussing personal issues take into consideration that person's dignity.**
- **The potential loss of independence can be threatening for some people.**
- **Offer to help a person to be able to see what problems they may be having.**
    - o **If they state they do not want help, as long as there are no safety concerns, allow them to perform the task by themselves.**

- When assisting someone, be sure their privacy is maintained.
- When events are planned, schedule an appropriate starting time so that the individual can do as much for themselves as possible in preparation of the event.

Possible outcomes:

- A poor outcome could cause a person to decline socializing if they are aware of their grooming challenges.
  - o General health can be adversely affected by lack of personal hygiene.
- A positive outcome includes cleanliness to maintain skin integrity and avoid infections.
  - o General health can be positively affected by personal hygiene.
- By allowing adequate time, and using assistive devices, independence may be maintained.

When to Call for Assistance:

- Consider asking for a referral for an occupational therapist to evaluate whether assistive devices may help an individual to remain independent in getting dressed, grooming, etc.
- Consider asking for a physical therapy evaluation if declining range of motion is being demonstrated.
- If a person does need assistance with personal care, there are many agencies that provide basic care.
  - o Working with that agency, try to find the best person who can provide care for an elderly individual.
    - ▪ Preferably this person has the skills and training for the care as well as a personality that blends with the elderly individual.

What the Doctor Needs to Know:

- **If there is concern that a person may be declining due to a health issue, such as an infection, be sure to seek advice from the person's primary health care provider.**

- **Since declining personal care may be a sign of depression be sure their health care provider is aware of changes in mood state or appearance.**

- **Discuss the need to have neuropsychological testing to determine a potential reason for a decline in personal care.**

  - o **The testing could help provide information about whether an individual needs increased supervision.**

Beerman, S., Rapport-Musson, J. (2002). *Eldercare 911.* Amherst, N.Y.: Prometheus Books.

National Institutes of Health. (2010). *Caregiver Guide: Tips for Caregivers of People with Alzheimer's Disease.* (NIH Publication No. 01-4013). Washington, DC: U. S. Government Printing Office.

Parkinson's Disease. (2012). In NIH online publication: *Senior Health.* Retrieved from: http://nihseniorhealth.gov/parkinsonsdisease/whatisparkinsonsdisease/01.html.

Robinson, A., White, L., Spencer, B. (2007) *Understanding Difficult Behaviors.* Ypsilanti, Michigan: Eastern Michigan University.

Chapter 17

THE TOPIC . . . . SKIN CARE

The Reason for the Topic:

- **Skin is the best defense from potential infections.**
- **Skin needs more attention as a person gets older because it becomes more fragile with age.**

Just a thought:

Deciphering skin rashes was never one my favorite things to do. But sometimes what looks like a rash is actually self-inflicted scratches.

Sometimes, we heard family members saying how they would try to prohibit scratching by attempting to persuade the individual to promise to quit.

This didn't solve the problem for several reasons. If a person has memory issues, it is likely they won't remember the agreement. Second, they will likely not remember to stop scratching. This ultimately causes a circle of arguments with little or no resolution to the original problem.

What helps more than anything is to remove the opportunity to scratch. Cover arms with sleeves. Also, have the person wear gloves. Then the individual can safely rub all they want to, but skin remains intact. If nothing else, these items provide a distraction.

Goals:

- Intact skin.
- No skin tears.
- Free of rashes.

Interventions:

- Observe skin whenever possible, e.g. while dressing or bathing.
- Don't use powder because it can clog pores.
  - o Use lotions that are easily absorbed and transparent.
- Avoid ointments that contain opaque white substances. If a rash develops under an opaque ointment, the rash can't be seen.
- For healthy skin, drink at least 6 glasses of water per day.
  - o If the outermost layer of skin is lightly pinched and it stays in a tent shape, dehydration is a concern.
- Be aware that fragile skin can tear easily.
  - o Simply by brushing past a door or removing clothing frail skin can tear.
- Have appropriate first aid bandages available in case of an injury. Keep the wound edges together to promote healing.
- For dry skin, try using a moisturizing lotion at bedtime. Then put gloves or a soft cloth over the lotion to help hold in the moisture.
- Observe for changes in moles.
- Refer to Chapter 1 for instructions when there are skin folds with redness or recurrent infections.

Possible outcomes:

- Positive outcomes include:
  - o Clear intact skin.
  - o No rashes.
  - o No infections.

- **Negative outcomes could include:**
  - o **Open wounds.**
  - o **Itching/scratching.**
  - o **Odors due to infections.**

When to Call for Assistance:

- **Read the labels on lotions prior to purchasing them.**
- **If it appears that someone may be allergic to a soap or lotion, consider seeking the advice of a dermatologist.**
- **Be sure to record changes in skin especially moles.**

What the Doctor Needs to Know:

- **If skin tears occur repeatedly be sure the health care provider is aware.**
- **Report all changes in moles, lesions, and rashes to the primary health care provider.**
- **Consider a referral to a dermatologist if skin issues become chronic concerns.**

Beerman, S., Rapport-Musson, J. (2002). *Eldercare 911.* Amherst, N.Y.: Prometheus Books.

National Institutes of Health. (2010). *Caregiver Guide: Tips for Caregivers of People with Alzheimer's Disease.* (NIH Publication No. 01-4013). Washington, DC: U. S. Government Printing Office.

Robinson, A., White, L., Spencer, B. (2007) *Understanding Difficult Behaviors.* Ypsilanti, Michigan: Eastern Michigan University.

Chapter 18

THE TOPIC . . . . SLEEP

The Reason for the Topic:

- Without restful sleep, people demonstrate challenges in concentration, mood state, and the ability to care for themselves.
    - o Walking around the room, taking a breath, and normal body functions use energy.
- Our system needs the recuperation that rest provides. Without quality sleep, rest cannot happen.
- Sleep apnea results from inadequate air flowing in and out of the lungs while a person is sleeping.
    - o If someone pauses to breathe during their sleep followed by a gasp or snoring type of breath, it may be obstructive sleep apnea.
    - o Various health concerns may result from untreated sleep apnea.
- Medications may cause a person to be unable to sleep.
    - o Even the medications that are intended to help a person get to sleep, may actually cause a sleep disturbance.
- Pain or lack of mobility due to an injury can prevent a person from finding a position of comfort.
    - o Without a comfortable position, sleep may be a challenge.

- **People who have been employed during regular night time sleeping hours for many years may not be able to adjust to sleeping at night.**
- **Restless leg syndrome causes unpredictable leg movements.**
  - o **People affected by restless leg syndrome notice their legs move whether they want them to or not.**

Just a thought:

Many people don't realize the full effects that restful sleep provides. However, if there is a cause for sleep disturbance, and it is corrected, the results can be amazing.

Without adequate rest, some people have demonstrated cognitive problems. If that person is over seventy or eighty years old, family members may be quick to think that the issue is dementia.

Frequently, at the Geriatric Assessment Clinic, our doctors would usually postpone cognitive testing until after sleep studies could rule out whether a sleep disorder may be the actual problem.

Goals:

- **Consistent sleeping pattern.**
- **Daytime wakefulness.**
- **Be better able to concentrate, problem solve, and plan.**
- **Basic bodily functions are able to meet the needs of day to day living due to a balance between active wakefulness and restful sleep.**

Interventions:

- **If someone is demonstrating sleep apnea, it is very important to notify their primary health care provider.**
  - o **A sleep study needs to be considered.**
- **Keeping a sleep log can be very helpful. Record the following information to discuss:**
  - o **Bedtime.**
  - o **How long it took to get to sleep.**
  - o **Number of times awake during the night.**

- o Number of times up to the bathroom.
- o Time of rising in the morning.
- o How the person felt upon rising.
  - Exhausted.
  - Rested.
  - Irritable.
- Discuss all the medications including prescription and over the counter medications with a pharmacist or your primary health care provider.
  - o Be sure to let them know about sleeping problems.
  - o Ask if any of the medications could be contributing to sleeping problems.
- Medications may be helpful to treat restless leg syndrome. Discuss this with the primary health care provider.
- Be sure the bedroom is a comfortable temperature.
- It is advisable to keep lighting minimal to aid in getting to sleep.
- Keep pets out of the bedroom when a person is trying to sleep.
- Be aware that some over the counter medications may cause sleep issues.

Possible outcomes:
- Best outcome is to wake up feeling rested.
- Improved daytime alertness.
- Worst outcome is an untreated sleep disorder that leads to serious health problems.

When to Call for Assistance:
- If a person is falling asleep in social settings, or multiple times throughout the day, lack of sleep needs to be discussed.
- If there have been changes in the person's wakefulness since medications have been changed, then keep a journal of this information to discuss with the health care provider.

- **If a person is taking over the counter medications, discuss the possibility of sleep problems due to those medications or supplements.**

What the Doctor Needs to Know:

- **If a person is experiencing sleep apnea:**
  - o **A pause in breathing followed by gasping for air or snoring.**
  - o **The health care provider needs to know this.**
  - o **Consider a sleep evaluation.**
- **If a person has fallen asleep while driving or even begins to nod, the health care provider also needs to know this.**
- **For anyone with difficulty sleeping and keeping a sleep log, be sure to bring the information to all health care appointments.**
- **Be sure to bring a list of all medications, including prescription and over the counter medications, to all appointments.**

Beerman, S., Rapport-Musson, J. (2002). *Eldercare 911.* Amherst, N.Y.: Prometheus Books.

National Institute on Aging. (2012). *Age Page: A Good Night's Sleep.* Washington, DC: U. S. Government Printing Office.

National Institute on Aging. (2013). *Age Page: Depression.* Washington, DC: U. S. Government Printing Office.

National Institute on Aging. (2014). *Alzheimer's Disease Medications.* (NIH Publication No. 08-3431). Washington, DC: U. S. Government Printing Office.

National Institutes of Health. (2010). *Caregiver Guide: Tips for Caregivers of People with Alzheimer's Disease.* (NIH Publication No. 01-4013). Washington, DC: U. S. Government Printing Office.

Robinson, A., White, L., Spencer, B. (2007) *Understanding Difficult Behaviors.* Ypsilanti, Michigan: Eastern Michigan University.

U. S. Department of Health and Human Services, National Institutes of Health. (2013). *Your Guide to Healthy Sleep.* (NIH Publication No. 11-5271.6) Washington, DC: U.S. Government Printing Office.

Chapter 19

THE TOPIC . . . . TEETH/ GUMS/MOUTH

The Reason for the Topic:

- Teeth are important for balanced nutrition.
- Teeth affect a person's appearance or their perception of their appearance.
- Healthy gums are essential for general health.
- Tooth or gum pain can be very debilitating, but preventable and treatable.

Just a thought:

I have said many times that the people I have cared for have taught me many lessons. One perspective had to do with dentures.

I remember asking a ninety year old gentleman if he had dentures or his own teeth. He promptly replied, "They're mine. I paid for them."

Then, I realized I needed to alter how I worded the question. After many possible options I chose to ask directly, "Do you have dentures?" Sometimes, I would ask more subtly whether their teeth were permanent.

Another lesson was learned when a lady instructed me that her teeth were "portable."

Goals:

- Able to chew without pain.
- No weight loss due to teeth and gum problems.
- No gum or tooth pain.
- No bad breath due to gum disease.

Interventions:

- Dental cleanings and checkups at least every 6 months.
- If someone has a partial, it is vital to have teeth and the partial checked routinely.
    - o If the partial becomes out of alignment with the teeth it uses as an anchor, it may result in the loss of more teeth.
- For anyone with complete dentures, it is important to have them checked at least every five years.
    - o Gradual changes may cause problems with gums. Preventive care is much less painful than treating sore gums.
    - o Also, not being able to wear dentures while the gums are healing can be an inconvenience.
- Routine brushing and flossing is the best way to keep teeth and gums in good health and appearance.
- For people who have difficulty flossing due to challenges with their dexterity, there are toothettes and other gum cleaning devices that may be more practical.
- Sometimes breathing through the mouth or certain medications may cause a coating of the tongue.
    - o Try mixing Milk of Magnesia with water or mouth wash using equal parts of each.
        - ▪ Coat the tongue with the mixture using toothette.
        - ▪ Wait about ten minutes then rinse with water or mouthwash.

- ▪ **Be sure not to swallow.**
- ▪ **Spit out the solution.**
- ▪ **Then rinse again.**

Possible outcomes:

- • **Positive outcomes include:**
  - o **Balanced nutrition as the result of positive oral maintenance.**
  - o **It feels good to smile.**
- • **Adverse outcomes include:**
  - o **Painful chewing.**
  - o **Weight loss due to painful chewing.**
  - o **Gum disease.**
  - o **Loss of teeth.**
  - o **Bad breath.**

When to Call for Assistance:

- • **Painful gums or chewing need to be addressed.**
- • **Contact a dentist if there is a chipped tooth that leaves a sharp edge.**
- • **Bleeding gums may be due to medications, dry mouth, or medical conditions.**
  - o **This needs to be reported to the health care provider.**
- • **Refusing to wear dentures due to pain may indicate the need for realignment.**

What the Doctor Needs to Know:

- • **The health care provider needs to be aware of any unexplainable weight loss.**
- • **If gums bleed with brushing or flossing, be sure your health care provider is aware.**

- **Be sure to visit the dentist routinely every six months for dental cleanings.**
- **For people with full dentures, they need to see a dentist at least every five years to check for alignment and excessive wear.**

Beerman, S., Rapport-Musson, J. (2002). *Eldercare 911*. Amherst, N.Y.: Prometheus Books.

National Institutes of Health. (2010). *Caregiver Guide: Tips for Caregivers of People with Alzheimer's Disease*. (NIH Publication No. 01-4013). Washington, DC: U. S. Government Printing Office.

Robinson, A., White, L., Spencer, B. (2007) *Understanding Difficult Behaviors*. Ypsilanti, Michigan: Eastern Michigan University.

Chapter 20

THE TOPIC .... VISION/EYES

The Reason for the Topic:

- Many safety issues are dependent on vision:
    - o Driving.
    - o Walking up and down stairs.
    - o Reading medication labels.
- Quality of life issues are impacted by changes in vision:
    - o Looking at pictures.
    - o Enjoying family moments.
    - o Reading.
- Some potential vision deficits are preventable.
- Some vision issues can be improved.
- Ignoring eye diseases could cause preventable blindness.

Just a thought:

Vision affects many dimensions of independent living. Quality of life can be worth the time and attention it takes to keep the senses as functional as possible. Many safety issues include the ability to see while driving, or reading, or walking to the bathroom.

I recall a number of people tell their stories of having cataracts removed. After surgery, they describe what clear vision is like. They can see things more vividly. The colors of their world announce the sights they had taken for granted.

Tending to the needs of eyes can take time and attention. But why neglect vision and potentially limit independence?

Goals:

- **Declining vision doesn't cause injuries to the person or others.**
- **Vision is optimal to enjoy family time and hobbies.**

Interventions:

- **Comprehensive vision assessment includes:**
  - o **Visual acuity.**
  - o **Check for cataracts.**
  - o **Assess for macular degeneration.**
  - o **Screening for glaucoma.**
  - o **Routine screenings at least every two years unless their findings conclude there is a problem.**
- **More frequent appointments are needed if a person is being monitored or treated for eye diseases.**
- **If you have Diabetes it is especially important to be aware of visual changes. Consider being evaluated by a retinal specialist.**

Possible outcomes:

- **Surgical removal of cataracts can restore vision that had become unclear due to cataracts.**

- Taking medications as directed can help keep Glaucoma from damaging visual fields.

  o Untreated Glaucoma can lead to tunnel vision and blindness.

- Retinal damage due to Diabetes can cause blindness.

- For anyone who is still driving, it is important to have routine eye exams.

When to Call for Assistance:

- Anyone with sudden loss of vision or eye pain call 911 or get to the nearest emergency room.

- If you notice someone holding a book very close to be able to read, they probably need to have their vision checked.

- If someone is avoiding glare, it may be due to glaucoma.

- If someone is tilting a page so they can look at it out of their side vision and not directly in front of them, they may have cataracts or macular degeneration.

What the Doctor Needs to Know:

- Be sure to keep a list of all eye drops on the list of medications for each appointment with the health care provider.

- Be sure to include all the eye drops you choose yourself, e.g. for dry eyes or itchy eyes.

- Be sure to have routine eye appointments with an ophthomologist.

Beerman, S., Rapport-Musson, J. (2002). *Eldercare 911*. Amherst, N.Y.: Prometheus Books.

National Institute on Aging. (2011) *Age Page: Aging and Your Eyes*. Washington, DC: U. S. Government Printing Office..

National Institutes of Health. (2010). *Caregiver Guide: Tips for Caregivers of People with Alzheimer's Disease*. (NIH Publication No. 01-4013). Washington, DC: U. S. Government Printing Office

SECTION 2

PROBLEMATIC BEHAVIORS

There are many perspectives to discussing problematic behaviors. Some behaviors are the result of psychological disorders. Medications sometimes contribute to changes in behavior.

Please note that the reason for the discussions of behavioral issues in the following chapters are for the sake of understanding some non-pharmacological approaches that caregivers can try. This is not intended to assist with prescribing medications or treating behaviors from a psychiatric perspective.

When it may be helpful, seeking medical or mental health advice is indicated.

Chapter 21

TOPIC . . . . APATHY

Just a thought:

I'm sure you have seen the look. A blank expression with no emotion to indicate any positive or negative thoughts or feelings. That's apathy. It's called a flat affect. It is also, a common symptom of depression or possibly advancing dementia.

Apathy can be described as not just a matter of not wanting to do something, but not wanting to want to. I have seen that expression on a number of nursing home residents. Then when activities are offered, so often they would respond, "No thank you."

However, if you simply took them to the activity, then suddenly those same individuals would start singing, or talking, or doing what everyone else was doing.

Apathy is not a disease, but it is a symptom that deserves attention.

Possible Causes:

- Dementia.
- Depression.
- Lack of sleep.
- Some medications.
- Lack of available socialization.
- Hearing loss.
- Visual impairment.

Possible dangers:

- If someone has untreated depression, avoidable apathy may occur.
- If someone is still driving, due to apathy they may be inattentive to their responsibilities. An automobile accident could result.
- Someone with apathy may not be aware of alarms or sounds around them that are intended to keep people safe.

Interventions:

- Someone demonstrating apathy needs to have a complete health assessment which may include:
  - o Vision.
  - o Hearing.
  - o Cognition.
  - o Depression screening.
  - o A medication review.
  - o A physical examination.
- Be sure social options are readily available.
- Keep a sleep log to assure adequate sleep is not the issue.
- Be sure medications are being taken correctly.

<u>When to call for help:</u>

- If the cause for apathy is known, become educated on that topic:
  - o If a person is diagnosed with a cognitive impairment, learn how best to approach the person's apathy.
  - o If a person's hearing is the issue, consider hearing aids or other devices.
  - o Be aware of extraneous background noises and distractions.
  - o If a person is not sleeping well, what are the causes?
    - How can their sleep be improved?
    - Is the person depressed?
    - What are the treatment options?
    - Does the person need changes in their environment?
    - Would fewer activities or the availability of more activities promote participation?
- Refer to Chapter 18 regarding sleep issues.
- Sometimes using a kind approach for suggestions is more readily accepted by an individual.
  - o In other words, don't state a list of options.
  - o It may be more useful to say, "It's time to go outside for a walk now."

<u>What the Doctor Needs to Know:</u>

- If a person has a sudden change in mood state, then be sure your primary health care provider is aware.
  - o Is the person less talkative?
  - o Is the person crying?
  - o Is the person withdrawn?
  - o Has the person stopped initiating self care?

- **If the health care provider makes suggestions, be sure to clarify the following:**
  - o **How long before the effectiveness is expected?**
  - o **What non-medication actions may be beneficial?**
  - o **If medications are ordered, what side effects might happen?**

Kalb, C. (2000). Coping with the Darkness: Revolutionary new approaches in providing care are helping people with Alzheimer's stay active and fe+el productive. *Newsweek*. (January).

National Institutes of Health. (2010). *Caregiver Guide: Tips for Caregivers of People with Alzheimer's Disease*. (NIH Publication No. 01-4013). Washington, DC: U. S. Government Printing Office.

Chapter 22

Topic . . . . AGITATION/ AGGRESSIVENESS/YELLING

Just a thought:

I recall that during my time as a nursing supervisor in a long term care unit, agitation was frequently demonstrated. Whenever a resident started to display behavior out of control, limiting escalation of the situation was one of the goals. Others residents who were nearby the occurrence were potentially in danger of injury, also.

Diversion could accomplish both goals. First, approach someone who has started to get loud and intense by using a pleasant voice. Then make a suggestion completely out of context. A person with short term memory loss might not be able to remember what caused their frustration.

Possible Causes:

- **There are many potential causes for agitated behavior.**
- **Some of the causes may include:**
    - o **Overtired.**
    - o **Bladder infection.**
    - o **Confusion due to dementia.**

- o Over stimulating environment.
- o Defensive perceptions.
- o Medication side effects.
- o Pain.
- o Post traumatic stress disorder.
- o Sun downing.

Possible dangers:

- The worst potential problems include injuries to the person and/or the caregivers.
  - o The individual could inadvertently be injured.
  - o The caregivers could get injured trying to care for the agitated person.
  - o Others nearby the incident could get injured.

Interventions:

- Be calm. Someone out of control will more likely escalate when they see someone else become irritable.
- Try not to rationalize with someone who is not oriented to time or place.
  - o They will only feel more insecure.
  - o This could cause them to become more anxious.
- Try to re-direct them.
  - o Use a positive/pleasant tone of voice.
  - o Choose a completely different topic in contrast to anything going on around the person.
    - Say in an upbeat tone, "I really like your pink shoes."
  - o Allow time for that person to be confused. More than likely they are processing information slowly. Do not try to rush or hurry an agitated individual to participate in a situation.

- If it is bath time, leave them alone and attempt bathing later.
- If it is meal time, leave them alone and attempt to provide food later.

  o When trying to re-direct a person, don't let the topic that caused agitation come back into the conversation if the individual is still upset.

  o Avoid touch until the person can recognize that you are not a threat to them.

  o When trying to re-direct them, if it doesn't work at first, allow time and space without jeopardizing the person themselves or others around them.

- Refer to Chapter 37 regarding sun downing.

When to call for help:

- Whenever a weapon is involved in an altercation, call 911.
- If a person is out of control and all options have been exhausted, then call 911 or take that individual to the nearest emergency room.
- Be advised that there are trainings for caregivers to learn how to handle agitated people.
- It is wise to become educated about how to avoid injuries to the individual as well as yourself and others.

What the Doctor Needs to Know:

- Keep a log of adverse behaviors.
  o Include the time of day.
  o What behaviors are occurring?
  o Are there any precipitating events?
  o What interactions have been tried?
- Ask if current medications could be causing increased agitation.

- **Discuss options for treating the behaviors:**
  - o **What non-pharmacological inventions may be helpful?**
  - o **What medications might be indicated?**

Beerman, S., Rapport-Musson, J. (2002). *Eldercare 911.* Amherst, N.Y.: Prometheus Books

National Institutes of Health. (2010). *Caregiver Guide: Tips for Caregivers of People with Alzheimer's Disease.* (NIH Publication No. 01-4013). Washington, DC: U. S. Government Printing Office.

Robinson, A., White, L., Spencer, B. (2007) *Understanding Difficult Behaviors.* Ypsilanti, Michigan: Eastern Michigan University.

Chapter 23

TOPIC . . . . ANXIETY

Just a thought:

There are times when people get up in the morning and sigh out loud, "What is there to worry about today?"

Then, with very little effort, there is usually some reason to fret. I was never sure if that helped to validate their plan to worry. Perhaps there could even be a sense of achievement due to their thought and preparation.

Anxiety doesn't need to deter congeniality or productivity. A person can also choose how to handle stress and may even worry less.

Possible Causes:

- **Lifelong anxiety.**
- **Stress.**
- **Lack of sleep.**
- **Depression.**
- **Certain medications.**
- **Caffeinated beverages.**

- Noisy environments.
- The need to multitask without adequate resources.

Possible dangers:
- Harm for the person or others.
- Loss of sleep.
- Poor nutritional choices.
- Poor safety choices.
- Distraction while performing routine tasks, e.g. driving, cooking, activities of daily living, etc.

Interventions:
- Write down times when anxiety occurs.
  o Include possible precipitating causes.
  o What behaviors have been witnessed, e.g. changes in respiration, wringing hands, ruminating, pacing, expressions?
- Try redirecting.
  o Use a calm voice.
  o Chose a topic appealing to the anxious person.
- If the environment is noisy or cluttered, try removing the person from that situation or altering the commotion.
- Limit all caffeine after noon.

When to call for help:
- If there is potential danger to the person or others, call 911.
- Attending support groups may provide mutually beneficial thoughts and ideas.
- Consider counseling.

<u>**What the Doctor Needs to Know**</u>:

- Be sure the primary health care provider is aware of all medications including any over the counter medications and supplements.

- Discuss whether current medications may be contributing to the anxiety symptoms.

- Discuss whether a medication may be beneficial.

- Take the notes describing the behaviors to all appointments with the health care provider.

- Discuss the option of meeting with a mental health professional.

Cowley, G. (2000). Alzheimer's Disease: Unlocking the Mystery. *Newsweek.* (January).

Robinson, A., White, L., Spencer, B. (2007) *Understanding Difficult Behaviors.* Ypsilanti, Michigan: Eastern Michigan University.

Chapter 24

TOPIC . . . . BOREDOM

Just a thought:

It never ceased to amaze me that when people moved into a nursing home, those who knew them very well believed they would just "give up."

Then within a few weeks, that same person who was thought to quietly sit and do nothing, started to participate in singing, and cooking, and social gatherings. When people are surrounded by others they can relate to, what might have looked like a decline in cognition or mood, may have simply been boredom.

Without initiative individuals may not realize how to keep themselves busy with hobbies or other tasks.

Possible Causes:

- Sometimes people are bored because there are simply no activities available for them.

- Apathy.

- Depression.

- Loss of skills to perform hobbies that were previously rewarding.

- Hearing loss decreasing the ability to interact with others.

- Dementia.
- Vision changes.

Possible dangers:

- Age doesn't mean a person can't participate in appropriate activities for their level of vision, hand skill, and thinking processes.
- When people stop doing things that brought them enjoyment their quality of life is also compromised.
- Lack of socializing could contribute to depression, apathy, and cognitive decline.

Interventions:

- Be sure to provide daily times for socializing with others.
- Get out of the house routinely even if it only involves getting into the car and driving around looking at scenery.
- Provide items for crafts if a person is still capable of doing hobby activities they have enjoyed.
- If a person has moderate to advanced dementia, allow them to fold clean laundry.
    o Dish towels and socks are good examples.

When to call for help:

- Senior Centers have varied activities that may provide a number of opportunities for participation and socialization.
- Find a program that provides senior companions.
- Participation in support groups may provide local options.

What the Doctor Needs to Know:

- Boredom is not a reason to medicate someone.
- Discuss the possibility that the person may be depressed.

Kalb, C. (2000). Coping with the Darkness: Revolutionary new approaches in providing care are helping people with Alzheimer's stay active and feel productive. *Newsweek.* (January).

National Institute on Aging. (2013). *Age Page: Depression.* Washington, DC: U. S. Government Printing Office.

National Institute on Aging. (2014) *Age Page: Exercise and Physical Activity: Getting Fit for Life.* Washington, DC: U. S. Government Printing Office.

Chapter 25

TOPIC . . . . CONFUSION

Just a thought:

As a person ages, it's not unusual to watch them slow down. Then it looks like they are becoming forgetful. The all too obviously conclusion is that they must have Alzheimer's Disease.

People may not want to know if they have dementia. But what if the real problem is a treatable condition? Wouldn't they want to know?

If the diagnosis of Alzheimer's Disease is confirmed, then options for treatment can be pursued. Second guessing confusion can only lead to . . . confusion.

Possible Causes:

- **Dementia is a progressive disease, but not the only reason an elderly person may be confused.**
- **Hypothyroid.**
- **Infections, especially bladder infections.**
    - o **Refer to Chapter 2 for further information about bladder infections.**
- **Lack of quality sleep. Refer to Chapter 18 regarding sleep issues.**
- **Depression.**

- Certain medications.
- Anemia.
- Pain.

Possible dangers:

- It would be unfortunate for a family to choose not to obtain diagnostic testing because they are convinced their loved one has Alzheimer's Disease. Later, the cause for the confusion was determined to be a treatable condition. It could have successfully been treated earlier if the incorrect assumption had not prevented diagnostic testing.
- People who are living alone are at a higher safety risk when they are confused.
    - o They could forget that they left the stove on and start a fire.
    - o They could forget to take their medications.
    - o They could forget to eat.
- They could forget to take care of themselves. e.g. personal care, possibly, lack of problem solving skills, or a potentially avoidable crisis.

Interventions:

- Seek medical attention to determine the cause of the confusion especially if the confusion appears to be a rapid decline.
- If there is a medical cause, then treatment is specific to that cause. (e.g. bladder infection, hypothyroid, anemia, etc.)
- If someone is frequently confused to time and date, it can increase their frustration to be quizzed about the date and time. Do not correct their errors.
- It may be helpful to post reminders that help a person but respects their privacy and dignity.

When to call for help:

- If a person is demonstrating changes in alertness and has a fever, the health care provider needs to be notified immediately.

What the Doctor Needs to Know:

- **Be sure to record what types of confusion a person has been demonstrating.**
  - o **Remembering names of their own children.**
  - o **Time of day.**
  - o **Getting lost.**
  - o **Confusing medication instructions.**
- **Bring the record to the next appointment with the health care provider.**
- **Discuss time of medication administration since some people have more difficulty in the late afternoon, or first thing in the morning.**

Beerman, S., Rapport-Musson, J. (2002). *Eldercare 911.* Amherst, N.Y.: Prometheus Books

National Institutes of Health. (2010). *Caregiver Guide: Tips for Caregivers of People with Alzheimer's Disease.* (NIH Publication No. 01-4013). Washington, DC: U. S. Government Printing Office.

National Institutes of Health. (2012). *Alzheimer's Disease; Fact Sheet.* (NIH Publication No. 11-6423). Washington, DC: U. S. Government Printing Office

Robinson, A., White, L., Spencer, B. (2007) *Understanding Difficult Behaviors.* Ypsilanti, Michigan: Eastern Michigan University.

Chapter 26

Topic . . . . DELUSIONS

Just a thought:

Sorting out truth from thoughts that cannot correlate with reality is not simple. Many delusions may sound reasonable. This could be due to the fact that the individual experiencing the delusional thinking, is completely convinced their statements are true.

For caregivers, assuring the safety of the individual and themselves is far more important than the lack of reality due to delusions.

Possible Causes:

- **Usually delusions are a mental health disorder.**
- **The causes and treatments for delusions are beyond the scope of this resource.**
- **The discussions here are for the purpose of helping caregivers to understand options for what to do or not to do.**

Possible dangers:

- **Delusions may cause a person to be dangerous to himself or others.**

Interventions:

- Referral to a behavioral specialist will be the most beneficial intervention.

- Arguing with the individual for the purpose of trying to convince them their thinking is wrong may only lead to increased frustration, anxiety, or escalate the situation beyond what it would be otherwise.

- Always be sure the person does not have access to items that they may use to injure themselves or others, e.g. remove weapons, car keys, knives, etc.

- Document the behaviors including:
  - Time of day?
  - What the person believes to be true?
  - What other behaviors the person is exhibiting, e.g. insomnia, anxiety, pacing, etc?
  - When did the delusion start?
  - Are there precipitating events or issues?
  - Are the delusions frightening to the individual?

When to call for help:

- If anyone is potentially in danger, call 911.

What the Doctor Needs to Know:

- Ask the primary health care provider if it would be helpful to have a psychological referral.

- Be sure to bring a list of behaviors when meeting with any health care professional.

- Always bring a list of all medications including over the counter medications to all health care appointments.

National Institute on Aging. (2014). *Age Page: Hallucinations, Delusions, and Paranoia: Alzheimer's Disease Caregiving Tips*. Washington, DC: U. S. Government Printing Office.

National Institutes of Health. (2010). *Caregiver Guide: Tips for Caregivers of People with Alzheimer's Disease*. (NIH Publication No. 01-4013). Washington, DC: U. S. Government Printing Office.

Robinson, A., White, L., Spencer, B. (2007) *Understanding Difficult Behaviors*. Ypsilanti, Michigan: Eastern Michigan University.

Chapter 27

Topic . . . .
EATING DISORDERS

Just a thought:

When a person doesn't feel hunger, it's challenging for them to want to eat. For an individual who is confused, distractions can swipe their attention away from their meal.

Aging presents enough challenges to balanced nutrition. Then add medical conditions and medications that upset the digestive process, and good nutrition should become a higher priority.

Possible Causes:

- **Eating disorders caused by psychological conditions are beyond the scope of this resource. However, the interventions discussed may be helpful for those situations.**

- **Typically, with the aging process the sense of smell diminishes and this can cause a decline in a person's appetite.**

- **Many medications effect how food tastes, which makes eating unappealing.**

- **Some medical problems cause a decline in appetite.**

- Depression can contribute to a decrease in motivation. Then people may be less likely to eat unless food is presented to them.

- As a person eats less for whatever reason, the digestive system produces less digestive enzymes. This causes a person to fill full sooner than they may have previously.

- Dental problems may cause a person to be reluctant to eat.

  o If teeth are loose, they may have trouble biting or chewing.

  o Painful gums could also affect an individual's ability to chew.

<u>Possible dangers</u>:

- Malnutrition.

- Adverse reactions to medications that need to be taken with food.

- Electrolyte imbalance due to poor fluid intake.

- Compromised healing ability.

- Weakened immune system.

<u>Interventions</u>:

- Dietary supplements need to be provided between meals.

  o If supplements are given with a meal, usually a person who needs the extra calories gets full too soon so they don't eat the meal.

  o Meals become an exchange of calories and not additional calories.

- Be sure a person is rested prior to meals. If a person is tired, they may not be motivated to eat.

- Avoid extra distractions during meal time.

- Some people cannot decide what they want to eat, but they will eat if food is placed in front of them.

  o If you know what foods they have always enjoyed, just simply serve it.

- If a person is depressed, it is kinder to not expect that individual to determine what to eat.

- If someone has been losing weight, be sure to weigh them routinely on the same scale, at the same time of day, wearing the same clothing.

- Keep a record of food and fluid intake.

- Refer to Chapter 19 regarding dental issues.

When to call for help:

- It may be helpful to seek a consultation with a dietician.

- Discussing medication and food interactions with a pharmacist may be helpful.

What the Doctor Needs to Know:

- Bring the following information to health care provider appointments:
  o Recorded weights.
  o Recorded intake.
  o List of all medications including prescription and over the counter medications.

- Ask the health care provider if any diagnostic studies would be helpful.

National Institute on Aging. (2014). *Alzheimer's Disease Medications*. (NIH Publication No. 08-3431). Washington, DC: U. S. Government Printing Office.

National Institutes of Health. (2010). *Caregiver Guide: Tips for Caregivers of People with Alzheimer's Disease*. (NIH Publication No. 01-4013). Washington, DC: U. S. Government Printing Office.

Robinson, A., White, L., Spencer, B. (2007) *Understanding Difficult Behaviors*. Ypsilanti, Michigan: Eastern Michigan University.

Chapter 28

TOPIC . . . . HALLUCINATIONS

Just a thought:

Individuals with Diffuse Lewy Body Disease frequently experience hallucinations. Many times the hallucinations aren't troubling to the person, then there are other times when the person becomes very distressed by what they see.

The main focus needs to always be the individual and their dignity.

Possible Causes:

- **Hallucinations are usually either a psychosis, a medical problem, or the result of a medication side effect. The purpose of this discussion is to help caregivers know what interactions to avoid, and to assist with understanding when to seek help.**

Possible dangers:

- **Hallucinations may cause a person to make potentially dangerous decisions.**
- **Hallucinations may become very disturbing to an individual.**

<u>Interventions:</u>

- Do not tell the person who is experiencing hallucinations that they are wrong.

- Respect the person who has hallucinations. Do not insinuate they are unintelligent or make them feel belittled.

- The most important intervention is for the primary health care provider to determine the cause for the hallucination. Then they need to decide either to treat or refer treatment to an appropriate specialist.

- Document the following characteristics of the hallucinations:

  o Are the hallucinations auditory or visual?

  o Is there a certain time of day hallucinations usually occur?

  o If they are visual, describe what the person states they see.

  o If they are auditory, describe what the person states they hear.

  o Are the hallucinations problematic to the individual?

  o Do they get scared?

  o Do they run outside due to the hallucinations?

<u>When to call for help:</u>

- When meeting with the primary health care provider, discuss the benefit of a mental health consultant.

<u>What the Doctor Needs to Know:</u>

- Be sure to bring the documentation of the hallucinations to all health care appointments.

- Ask the health care provider whether there is a medical reason for the hallucinations.

- Ask the health care provider whether medication is causing the hallucinations.

National Institute on Aging. (2014) *Talking with Your Doctor: A Guide for Older People.* (NIH Publication No. 05-3452). Washington, DC: U.S. Government Printing Office

National Institute on Aging. (2014). *Age Page: Hallucinations, Delusions, and Paranoia: Alzheimer's Disease Caregiving Tips.* Washington, DC: U. S. Government Printing Office.

National Institute on Aging. (2014). *Alzheimer's Disease Medications.* (NIH Publication No. 08-3431). Washington, DC: U. S. Government Printing Office.

National Institutes of Health. (2014). *Lewy Body Dementia: Information for Patients, Families, and Professionals.* (NIH Publication 13-7907). Washington, DC: U. S. Government Printing Office.

Parkinson's Disease. (2012). In NIH online publication: *Senior Health.* Retrieved from: http://nihseniorhealth.gov/parkinsonsdisease/whatisparkinsonsdisease/01.html.

Robinson, A., White, L., Spencer, B. (2007) *Understanding Difficult Behaviors.* Ypsilanti, Michigan: Eastern Michigan University.

Chapter 29

Topic . . . . HIDING THINGS

Just a thought:

It's natural to want to protect your own things. But when short term memory loss prevents a person from remembering where they put things, then frustration results.

At times families perceive their loved one as lying when they can't find things. People need to realize that it takes a fairly high functioning person to plan how and where to hide things. Usually, a person with dementia isn't capable of the multiple step organizing to accomplish a purposeful mission of hiding things then blaming others.

Accepting an individual's limitations can be the first step to avoid frustration. Realize the disease is at fault, not the person.

Possible Causes:

- **When a person has dementia, they may try to use their limited logic to protect themselves and their belongings.**

- **Some people try to place things in that one place where they will be sure to remember where they put it, but then can't remember where that special place was.**

- Short term memory loss.
- Impaired executive functioning.

Possible dangers:
- If things are inadvertently hidden that may have consequences later, e.g. the phone, car keys, important papers, etc.
- Anxiety or frustration can result from not finding something.
- Frustration and mistrust could result from an inability to accept that the hidden item wasn't stolen.

Interventions:
- If a person with dementia is hiding things, the first thing to know is what not to do:
  o Do not accuse the person of anything.
  o Do not expect the person to explain why things are being hidden.
  o Do not demonstrate frustration or anger toward the person.
  o Do not tell them they must remember where things are.
- Interactions that might be helpful.
  o "Let's look together."
  o "It can be replaced."
  o "Let's think about something else."
- If a person is totally frustrated, change the subject by using diversion.
- If objects that are repeatedly "hidden" or "lost" replace them with items that are larger and more difficult to be hide, e.g. if a women repeated loses or hides her purse, buy one too large to hide.
- Try not to demonstrate frustration even if it is a stressful situation.

When to call for help:
- Participating in support groups can help the caregiver to learn how others in similar situations are handling hiding things.

<u>What the Doctor Needs to Know:</u>

- **There is no medication to specifically treat hiding things, but it is helpful for the primary health care provider to be aware of all behavior changes.**

- **Discuss medication options for treating dementia.**

- **Neuropsychological testing to determine cognitive impairment.**

Cowley, G. (2000). Alzheimer's Disease: Unlocking the Mystery. *Newsweek.* (January).

National Institutes of Health. (2010). *Caregiver Guide: Tips for Caregivers of People with Alzheimer's Disease.* (NIH Publication No. 01-4013). Washington, DC: U. S. Government Printing Office.

National Institutes of Health. (2012). *Alzheimer's Disease; Fact Sheet.* (NIH Publication No. 11-6423). Washington, DC: U. S. Government Printing Office.

Chapter 30

Topic . . . . HOARDING

Just a thought:

Hoarding can be a serious safety concern. If quantities of stored items prohibit a person from exiting their house in case of a fire, the situation could potentially be life threatening.

Making home visits for the Geriatric Assessment Clinic I entered the homes of many hoarders. Newspapers, gum wrappers, egg cartons, etc., filled many rooms. Sometimes there was only a narrow trail to find the next room.

However, the individual's dignity is not unimportant. Approaching the situation in a timely way can support both the safety needs and the emotional status of the person.

Possible Causes:

- **Hoarding can be a pathological disease. The purpose of this discussion is not to analyze and treat hoarding. This information is intended to help caregivers realize safety concerns associated with hoarding.**

Possible dangers:

- There are many safety concerns including limiting potential exits due to quantity of items in front of exit doors and escape windows.

  o This could cause problems in case of a fire.

- Unsanitary living conditions when hoarding includes items that result in infestations.

- Clutter could potentially cause falls.

Interventions:

- Seek professional behavioral health personnel to discuss options for understanding, supporting, and working with a hoarder.

- Realize that safety issues are important reasons to not delay seeking assistance with hoarding.

When to call for help:

- Attending support groups may be helpful.

- It may be necessary to contact protective services.

What the Doctor Needs to Know:

- Discuss the option of a mental health consultation.

Beerman, S., Rapport-Musson, J. (2002). *Eldercare 911.* Amherst, N.Y.: Prometheus Books.

National Institutes of Health. (2010). *Caregiver Guide: Tips for Caregivers of People with Alzheimer's Disease.* (NIH Publication No. 01-4013). Washington, DC: U. S. Government Printing Office.

Chapter 31

TOPIC . . . . INAPPROPRIATE SOCIAL BEHAVIORS

Just a thought:

Participating in social events needs to be a routine part of life. Socializing helps mood, memory, and motivation. It provides a positive quality to daily living.

However, if a person can no longer control their behavior embarrassing situations can result. Intervening to protect the individual and others from emotional and physical injury needs to be a priority.

Possible Causes:

- Frontal lobe dementias tend to have more pronounced socially inappropriate behaviors, e.g. Picks Disease, Frontotemporal Dementia, etc.

- As cognitive functions decline, a person with any type of dementia can develop an inability to maintain socially acceptable skills and habits.

Possible dangers:

- Due to embarrassment or confrontational situations, people may potentially become vulnerable to unpredictable consequences.

Interventions:

- Avoid situations where impulsive behaviors could be disruptive, e.g. congested public places.
- Realize that a person's behavior is the result of a disease process and is not the fault of the person.
  - o It is the fault of the disease.
- Be prepared to redirect a person if they cause an embarrassing moment.
- Do not avoid all socialization for a person who demonstrates inappropriate social behavior.
- Be sure to establish and maintain appropriate boundaries.

When to call for help:

- Attending support groups may help understand the individual's behavior and hear what others share about similar challenges.
- It may be helpful to seek professional guidance to learn how to establish boundaries.

What the Doctor Needs to Know:

- Discuss all behaviors with primary health care providers.
- It is important to know that there are no medications to treat social skills.

National Institutes of Health. (2014). *Frontotemporal Disorders: Information for Patients, Families, and Caregivers.* (NIH Publication No. 14-6361). Washington, DC: U. S. Government Printing Office.

Beerman, S., Rapport-Musson, J. (2002). *Eldercare 911.* Amherst, N.Y.: Prometheus Books.

Robinson, A., White, L., Spencer, B. (2007) *Understanding Difficult Behaviors.* Ypsilanti, Michigan: Eastern Michigan University.

National Institutes of Health. (2010). *Caregiver Guide: Tips for Caregivers of People with Alzheimer's Disease.* (NIH Publication No. 01-4013). Washington, DC: U. S. Government Printing Office.

Chapter 32

Topic . . . . INSOMNIA

Just a thought:

It doesn't seem possible, but on many occasions I have seen this happen. A person with Alzheimer's Disease doesn't sleep for three continuous days and nights. No caregiver can keep up with that routine no matter what.

"He hasn't slept since Tuesday!" We have heard this statement repeatedly. "I don't know what keeps him going!"

No one else does either. Remember, no one is endangered due to insomnia unless they wander into an unsafe situation. Often once a person does sleep, they are awake again for several days.

There is no other word than respite. One solution is to have the adult children take turns with the parent who needs supervision, so the other parent can rest. If the caregiver doesn't get adequate rest, the situation becomes a safety issue for them.

Possible Causes:

- **Caffeine.**
- **Certain medications may contribute to insomnia. Sometimes medications originally directed to be given at bedtime, actually cause sleep disturbances.**

o But for some people it caused vivid dreams so rest was not accomplished if the person slept. Some people couldn't sleep.

- Some people with dementia simply do not sleep very much.

Possible dangers:
- If a person is unsupervised, they may wander outside. That would be potentially very dangerous.
- If a person is unsupervised they may injure themselves or fall.
- If a caregiver tries to provide all the supervision with inadequate sleep, this is unsafe for both the person and the caregiver.
- Caregiver burnout will happen unless the they will allow respite or help. The general health of the caregiver could be unnecessarily at risk.

Interventions:
- Avoid allowing a person to sleep more than an hour during the day. Sleeping during day can cause a person not be drowsy at bedtime.
- Avoid caffeine especially after noon.
- Maintain a bedtime routine to promote sleep.
- Avoid extra stress or activity during the evening.
- Be sure the bedroom is a comfortable temperature.
- Have adequate lighting to prevent falls if someone needs to get up, but dimly lit to promote sleep.
- Consider keeping pets out of the bedroom.
- Refer to Chapter 18 for additional information regarding sleep.

When to call for help:
- It is wise for a caregiver to arrange assistance and respite prior to becoming so tired they stop taking care of their own needs.
- If someone cannot meet their own needs, then it becomes more challenging to take of care of their loved.

What the Doctor Needs to Know:

- **Be sure the primary health care provider is aware of sleep issues.**

- **Discuss whether the medications may be contributing to the insomnia.**

- **Do the times of the medications need to be adjusted?**

U. S. Department of Health and Human Services, National Institutes of Health. (2013). *Your Guide to Healthy Sleep*. (NIH Publication No. 11-5271.6) Washington, DC: U.S. Government Printing Office.

National Institute on Aging. (2012). *Age Page: A Good Night's Sleep*. Washington, DC: U. S. Government Printing Office.

Robinson, A., White, L., Spencer, B. (2007) *Understanding Difficult Behaviors*. Ypsilanti, Michigan: Eastern Michigan University.

National Institutes of Health. (2010). *Caregiver Guide: Tips for Caregivers of People with Alzheimer's Disease*. (NIH Publication No. 01-4013). Washington, DC: U. S. Government Printing Office.

Chapter 33

TOPIC . . . . PHYSICALLY ABUSIVE

Just a thought:

Dementia is never a reason to accept physical assault. If a person is out of control to the point that physical abuse is occurring, this is unacceptable. Calling for assistance to intervene is vital.

Inappropriate body contact can result in not only physical pain, but emotional pain, also.

As dementia progresses, a person's ability to make appropriate reactions to situations may decline. It is rarely a possibility to rationalize with an individual with dementia. Once a person is out of control physically, it becomes less likely that trying to discuss or negotiate with that person will resolve the situation. It may only cause their behavior to escalate.

Possible Causes:

- **Life long history of abuse, either being abused, or causing abuse.**
- **Post traumatic stress disorder.**
- **Inadequate stress management skills.**
- **Lack of anger management skills.**
- **Frontotemporal Dementia.**
- **Some mental health disorders.**

Possible dangers:

- Injury to the caregiver.
- Injury to the individual.
- Injury to an individual confronted by the abusive person.
- Emotional damage as a result of being abused.

Interventions:

- If someone is out of control and presenting a physical threat, call 911.
- Caregivers need to protect themselves and remove themselves from harm.
- People with dementia should not have access to firearms or other weapons.
- Seek help from professionals who are trained to work with people/families in abusive situations.

When to call for help:

- If anyone is assaulted, call 911.
- If there is an abusive situation, protective services needs to be consulted.
- Attending support groups may be helpful to learn guidelines for boundaries and assuring safety for everyone.
- Seek counseling.

What the Doctor Needs to Know:

- Be sure that the health care provider is aware of aggressive behaviors.
- Discuss options for consultations with mental health professionals.

National Institutes of Health. (2010). *Caregiver Guide: Tips for Caregivers of People with Alzheimer's Disease.* (NIH Publication No. 01-4013). Washington, DC: U. S. Government Printing Office.

National Institutes of Health. (2012). *Alzheimer's Disease; Fact Sheet.* (NIH Publication No. 11-6423). Washington, DC: U. S. Government Printing Office.

Robinson, A., White, L., Spencer, B. (2007) *Understanding Difficult Behaviors.* Ypsilanti, Michigan: Eastern Michigan University.

Chapter 34

Topic . . . . REFUSING CARE

Just a thought:

There were times I was concerned about elderly people living alone. When someone would refuse to eat, bathe, take their medications, etc., it caused concern whether they were safe.

Independence is an understandable goal. But sometimes, having a certain amount of assistance, can actually provide the opportunity for an individual to remain in their own home.

Possible Causes:

- **As dementia progresses, it is common for a person to have no insight regarding their limitations.**

- **If a person refuses bathing it may be due to an adverse experience when they younger.**
    - o **Sometimes people who had a near drowning experience, are frightened to bathe or shower.**
    - o **Refer to Chapter 1.**

- **Sometimes people try to maintain independence because they are unaware of their declining cognition.**
    - o **Without realizing it, they jeopardize their safety.**

Possible dangers:

- If a person is not taking care of themselves, and also refuses to accept care from others, but still lives alone, they may be seriously endangering themselves.

- If a person who still uses the stove or oven, doesn't remember to turn it off, a fire may start.

- If a person is hearing impaired, and refuses to wear hearing aids, they may not hear a smoke alarm.

- A person who is cognitively impaired may not be able to problem solve situations like what to do if there is a power outage.

- If an individual is refusing to bathe they are at risk for infections and body odor.

Interventions:

- When an elderly person is alone and potentially endangered protective services may need to be involved to assess the situation.

- It may be imperative to remove the knobs from the stove and oven if there is a chance that a fire could be inadvertently started.

- A person with memory loss cannot be held responsible for remembering what to do or not do.
  - o If a family is aware that their loved one cannot care for themselves and that person is not competent, then it is the responsibility of the family to assure their safety.

- Respecting a person's dignity while asserting that their care is accomplished could include:
  - o Try using diversion to dissuade their refusal.
  - o Provide adequate privacy.
  - o If bathing is an issue, be sure the room is warm, and use the simplest tactics. Explain one step at a time.
  - o Seek to find ways that do not cause frustration for the person. Attempt to bathe at different times of the day.

- Refer to Chapter 1.
  o Even if it takes longer to accomplish a task, allow the person to perform as much self care as they can do safely.
    - Refer to Chapter 16.

When to call for help:

- If a person is in imminent danger, call 911.

- If person is living alone and is not safe, consider contacting protective services.

- Attending support groups with others who face the same challenges may be helpful.

- Consider hiring an agency to assist the person in their own home.

What the Doctor Needs to Know:

- If cognitive testing has not been done, at this time cognitive testing would help identify whether the person is competent to make their own decisions.

- Cognitive testing will also help identify what types of supervision an individual needs, e.g. cooking, medications, handling finances, driving, as well as living alone.

- This information will be helpful for protective services' staff to determine a person's independence capabilities.

National Institutes of Health. (2010). *Caregiver Guide: Tips for Caregivers of People with Alzheimer's Disease.* (NIH Publication No. 01-4013). Washington, DC: U. S. Government Printing Office.

Robinson, A., White, L., Spencer, B. (2007) *Understanding Difficult Behaviors.* Ypsilanti, Michigan: Eastern Michigan University.

Zarit, S. H., Zarit, J. M. (2007) *Mental Disorders in Older Adults.* (2nd ed.) New York: The Guilford Press.

Chapter 35

TOPIC . . . . REFUSING TO CHANGE CLOTHING

Just a thought:

Sometimes things are too obvious. A wife would complain that her husband always put on the same clothes day after the day.

The logical question was where he put his clothes at the end of the day? If the answer was that he put them back in the closet, then the solution seemed rather obvious.

Remove the clothes from his closet and place them in the washing machine.

Possible Causes:

- **As dementia progresses it is common for a person to lack insight to their own needs or abilities.**

Possible dangers:

- **Lack of adequate hygiene can lead to skin problems, infections, rashes, and body odor.**

- **Disheveled appearance can have an adverse effect in social settings.**

Interventions:

- Remove previously worn clothing. Place them out of sight possibly in the washing machine directly.

- Place clean clothes readily available for the person to dress themselves.

- If a battle results from the suggestion to remove clothing, further agitation may result.

  o **Refer to Chapter 22.**

- Remember that the sense of smell dissipates over time. Because that happens, people with significant body odor do not usually smell their own body odor.

- Appearance is a dignity issue. Deliberately trying to embarrass someone to force them to change their clothes is demeaning and rarely effective.

When to call for help:

- Attending support groups may be helpful to share stories with others who are challenged by similar behaviors.

- Sometimes individuals will accept help with personal care from a trained agency assistant more readily than from family members.

What the Doctor Needs to Know:

- If there has not been a discussion with the health care provider about establishing a cognitive diagnosis, this would be the time.

- If declining self care efforts are due to dementia, then initiating an appropriate medication may help.

National Institutes of Health. (2010). *Caregiver Guide: Tips for Caregivers of People with Alzheimer's Disease.* (NIH Publication No. 01-4013). Washington, DC: U. S. Government Printing Office.

Robinson, A., White, L., Spencer, B. (2007) *Understanding Difficult Behaviors.* Ypsilanti, Michigan: Eastern Michigan University.

Chapter 36

TOPIC . . . . REPETITIVE BEHAVIORS

Just a thought:

I have seen many residents in a nursing home, repeat behaviors. The only ones who seem bothered by the behavior are their family members. As they watch their loved one, they try to figure out how to stop the behavior.

Perhaps what might be more useful, is to try to understand that the behavior may bring comfort and a sense of control to the individual.

Possible Causes:
- Sometimes repetitive behaviors provide a sense of security.
- There may be a psychological reason. The scope of this chapter is not to pursue psychoses, but to know how to keep a person safe.

Possible dangers:
- If any behavior endangers a person or others, consider calling 911.

Interventions:
- Depending on the type of repetitive behavior, provide a safe environment.

- o **If someone washes their hands repeatedly, have soap available that is not harsh to skin. Also, offer lotion frequently for the person to massage into their hands.**
- o **If a person's repetitive behavior causes others to become irritated, the individual may need to be removed from that situation.**
- **Be advised that attempting to stop a person from repetitive behaviors may cause anxiety. If there is no danger to the person or others, consider allowing the behavior to continue.**

When to call for help:

- **It may be helpful to seek professional help from a behavioral health specialist to understand the behavior and know how to respond.**

What the Doctor Needs to Know:

- **Record all behaviors to discuss with the health care provider.**
- **Discuss the benefit of a mental health consultation.**

Kalb, C. (2000). Coping with the Darkness: Revolutionary new approaches in providing care are helping people with Alzheimer's stay active and feel productive. *Newsweek*. (January).

National Institute on Aging. (2013). *Age Page: Depression*. Washington, DC: U. S. Government Printing Office.

Robinson, A., White, L., Spencer, B. (2007) *Understanding Difficult Behaviors*. Ypsilanti, Michigan: Eastern Michigan University.

Chapter 37

TOPIC . . . . SUN DOWNING

Just a thought:

We heard the story many times. The person would be fine all day. Then between 2:30 pm and 4:00 pm things would change. The first signs may have been subtle. Then a predictable escalation of anxiety occurs with louder vocal objections to anything and everything. The sun downing begins.

The same time of day, similar behavior, and predictable changes are trademarks for problem behavior. However predictable it seems, sun downing can be a caregiver's challenge.

The best treatment seems to be to avoid the chain reaction from the start. Once the process starts, redirecting the agitation seems nearly impossible to deter.

As the sun sets, so does the calm.

Possible Causes:

- **Sun downing happens frequently to people with dementia.**

- **Mid to late afternoon a person's agitated behavior begins or escalates and is very difficult to redirect.**

- **The precise cause is unknown, but being over tired may contribute to the behaviors.**

<u>Possible dangers:</u>

- If a person becomes extremely out of control they can become a danger to themselves or others.

- If a person tries to leave due to their behavior, the consequences of going outside could be dangerous.

<u>Interventions:</u>

- It can be helpful to document the following details. Studying patterns and trends of someone exhibiting sun downing may provide clues regarding what is causing the problem and what might help:
    - What time does the behavior usually start?
    - What was happening in the environment prior to the behavior, e.g. noisy, lots of people, commotion, etc.?
    - What type of behavior is exhibited, e.g. yelling, kicking, pacing, threatening, delusions, etc.?
    - What efforts have been tried to avoid the occurrence, e.g. resting after lunch, minimizing noise, quiet environment, etc.?
    - What medications have been used and were the results effective, slightly effective, or ineffective?

- If a person's sun downing behavior begins to escalate and is not a danger to themselves or others, it is acceptable to stay back and let them have a time to unwind.
    - Usually, the sun downing behavior is self-limiting.
    - Too much attention could make the situation more intense.

- Consider respite for family caregivers who can become fatigued by loved ones who demonstrate sun downing.

<u>When to call for help:</u>

- If the situation becomes dangerous, call 911.

- Support groups for caregivers may be helpful to hear and share similar experiences.

What the Doctor Needs to Know:

- Take the behavior log to appointments with health care providers.

- Be sure to bring a list of all medications to all health care appointments. This includes prescription medications as well as over the counter medications and supplements.

Beerman, S., Rapport-Musson, J. (2002). *Eldercare 911*. Amherst, N.Y.: Prometheus Books.

National Institutes of Health. (2010). *Caregiver Guide: Tips for Caregivers of People with Alzheimer's Disease*. (NIH Publication No. 01-4013). Washington, DC: U. S. Government Printing Office.

Robinson, A., White, L., Spencer, B. (2007) *Understanding Difficult Behaviors*. Ypsilanti, Michigan: Eastern Michigan University.

Chapter 38

Topic . . . . VERBALLY ABUSIVE

Just a thought:

In the nursing home, there were a number of residents who could become threatening toward staff not to mention other residents. Keeping everyone safe and calm was always the goal.

Sometimes short term memory loss can be an advantage. Try to use a light hearted compliment directed to the one being verbally hurtful. This might surprise them. Then, follow the distraction with a completely different topic. The angry person may not remember what upset them.

Possible Causes:

- **Lifelong behaviors of being abused and abusing others.**
- **Anxiety/depression.**
- **Lack of sleep.**
- **Environment of excessive commotion.**
- **Poor stress management skills.**
- **Poor anger management skills.**

Possible dangers:

- Yelling that escalates can potentially result in injury to the person or others.
- Emotional damage.

Interventions:

- If a situation is out of control, consider calling 911.
- Redirect the current topic.
    o Use a nonthreatening tone of voice.
    o Attempt to alter the environment to decrease commotion.
- If the person is high enough functioning to understand, then state clearly that their behavior is unacceptable.
- Be aware that rationalizing may cause a person's behavior to escalate.
- Attempt to set boundaries to prevent escalating of the situation.
- Be advised that a person with advancing dementia may not have the cognitive ability to realize what they are saying or the result of their words.
- If possible, remove vulnerable people from the situation.

When to call for help:

- If the situation becomes threatening, call 911.
- Consider contacting protective services.
- Consider counseling to learn how to understand and set boundaries.
- Attending support groups may provide practical examples how others are handling similar challenges.
- Caregivers need to understand they should remove themselves from physically abusive situations.

What the Doctor Needs to Know:

- Make a list of adverse behaviors and bring to appointments with the health care provider.

- **Consider discussing a referral to a behavioral health specialist.**

- **Medications don't generally change personality behaviors, but if the behavior is caused by a treatable health issue this should be discussed with the health care provider.**

National Institutes of Health. (2010). *Caregiver Guide: Tips for Caregivers of People with Alzheimer's Disease.* (NIH Publication No. 01-4013). Washington, DC: U. S. Government Printing Office.

National Institutes of Health. (2012). *Alzheimer's Disease; Fact Sheet.* (NIH Publication No. 11-6423). Washington, DC: U. S. Government Printing Office.

National Institutes of Health. (2014). *Frontotemporal Disorders: Information for Patients, Families, and Caregivers.* (NIH Publication No. 14-6361). Washington, DC: U. S. Government Printing Office.

Robinson, A., White, L., Spencer, B. (2007) *Understanding Difficult Behaviors.* Ypsilanti, Michigan: Eastern Michigan University.

Robinson, A., White, L., Spencer, B. (2007) *Understanding Difficult Behaviors.* Ypsilanti, Michigan: Eastern Michigan University.

Chapter 39

Topic . . . . WANDERING

Just a thought:

I couldn't begin to recall the vast array of wandering stories that I have witnessed in my thirty years as a gerontological nurse. People would climb out of bed in the middle of the night and roam the hallways for hours. Others, seemed determined to go outside no matter what the weather was doing.

Families also told stories of their loved ones walking from one room to another. Probably the kindest lesson to be learned, is simple safety.

If the person is content to wander within a certain part of the home, and they are not in any danger, there is nothing wrong with wandering.

Many families would comment to the Geriatric Assessment Clinic team that their concern was wandering. Dementia causes a number of concerns, but wandering may not be a problem depending on the situation.

Possible Causes:

- **A person with short term memory loss may not recognize their current surroundings and feel the need to go somewhere else.**

- **It is nearly impossible to know what a person with dementia is thinking and why they make the decisions they do.**

- o Sometimes they may be reminded of something a long time ago and feel the need to leave.
- Sometimes people feel the need to get up and go.
  - o They simply have no idea where are going.
  - o Their wandering does not have any specific purpose.

Possible dangers:

- If people wander at night, they my wander out into cold weather and not realize it. They are at risk for hypothermia, frost bite, or even death.
- Wandering away and not being able to find their way back.
  - o They could get lost.
- If people who live in a city wander outside, they are at a higher risk of getting hit by a vehicle.

Interventions:

- Install alarms on the doors.
- Allow a person to be ambulatory in a safe setting.
- As long as a person is not endangering himself or others, there is no reason wandering needs to stop. Keeping people mobile is healthy for a number of reasons.
  - o Refer to Chapter 12.
- Block stairways so that a wandering person does not inadvertently fall down the stairs.
- Be advised that wandering is not a reason to medicate a person. Medications will not stop wandering, but may cause a person to become groggy and have a higher risk of falling.
- When a caregiver is responsible for a person who wanders, they need respite.
  - o It can be exhausting to supervise, observe, and care for a wanderer.

When to call for help:

- If someone is missing or in danger, call 911.

- Attending support groups to hear what others have done in their situations can be helpful.

- If someone is a night time wanderer, consider hiring someone to be awake during those hours to provide supervision so that the primary caregiver can get adequate rest.

- Discuss wandering behaviors with adult children to determine how they may be able to assist with supervision.

- Consider obtaining a global positioning device for the individual to wear in case they wander away from home.

What the Doctor Needs to Know:

- Keep a list of concerns to discuss at the appointments with health care providers.

National Institutes of Health. (2010). *Caregiver Guide: Tips for Caregivers of People with Alzheimer's Disease.* (NIH Publication No. 01-4013). Washington, DC: U. S. Government Printing Office.

National Institutes of Health. (2012). *Alzheimer's Disease; Fact Sheet.* (NIH Publication No. 11-6423). Washington, DC: U. S. Government Printing Office.

Robinson, A., White, L., Spencer, B. (2007) *Understanding Difficult Behaviors.* Ypsilanti, Michigan: Eastern Michigan University.

Chapter 40

TOPIC .... WANTING TO GO HOME

Just a thought:

I have witnessed people stand in their own living room that was built by their own hands, and ask to "go home." Residents in nursing homes may pack their belongings routinely preparing to go home, even though the plan is for them to stay.

It may be easy to think about that feeling of warmth when as a child a person comes in from a snowy day. Their mom makes hot cocoa with little tiny marshmallows. It's called comfort. It's called safety.

Most people asking to go home, don't know how to ask for safety and comfort, but that is what they are saying.

Possible Causes:

- **Usually, people who repeatedly ask to go home are individuals with at least moderately advanced dementia.**

- **A sense of safety is important at any stage of life. It is possible that a person asking to "go home" is not actually referring to their current home, but rather a place of safety and security when they were much younger.**

Possible dangers:

- Stress may increase for caregivers when their loved one repeatedly makes requests that cannot be satisfied. Asking to go home frequently may be a source of frustration for the caregiver.

- When a person does not understand their own needs, meeting that person's expectation becomes more difficult if not impossible. This adds to the caregiver burdens.

Interventions:

- Use the word "safe" repeatedly.

- Try not to rationalize. Telling someone, "You are home," seems like a conflict to the individual who is asking to go home.

- Offer non-threatening touch to the hand, arm, or shoulder.

- Use a soft tone of voice.

- Re-direct the person to a completely different topic they enjoy.

When to call for help:

- Attending support groups you will hear how others have been dealing with the same challenges.

- Also, sharing your situation at support groups may help others.

- If there is a chance of injury to the person or caregiver, call 911.

What the Doctor Needs to Know:

- Be sure that the health care provider is aware of all behaviors.

National Institutes of Health. (2010). *Caregiver Guide: Tips for Caregivers of People with Alzheimer's Disease.* (NIH Publication No. 01-4013). Washington, DC: U. S. Government Printing Office.

Robinson, A., White, L., Spencer, B. (2007) *Understanding Difficult Behaviors.* Ypsilanti, Michigan: Eastern Michigan University.

SECTION 3

A WALK THROUGH THE HOUSE

Many people live with the plan to stay in their own home for as long as possible. Sometimes as individuals age, they don't always realize their declining skills.

The following chapters discuss potential concerns specific to different parts of a home. Included in the chapters are examples of various situations that I witnessed during my years as a gerontological nurse.

So now, let's take . . . . . A Walk Through the House.

Chapter 41

AREA OF THE HOUSE . . . .
THE ADDRESS NUMBER

Potential Safety issues:

- **If emergency vehicles are trying to find your home, is the address number easy to see from the road or street in front of your house?**

Just a thought:

I could tell you many entertaining moments in trying to locate places when I was performing home visits as a nurse. In recent years, I have become dependent on electronic mapping devices. But in the early years, sometimes the only way to find the location of someone I was scheduled to visit was to ask them for directions.

Hearing directions that included information like "turn right at the one room school house," or "watch for the house that looks like a barn, then turn left, after the next road." This sounded like directions that should have been helpful, except for the fact that I turned at the wrong one room school house. Plus, the definition of a house looking like a barn is a little subjective.

The directions I found the most intriguing were when someone would say, "Turn at the tree."

This led me to ask, "What tree?"

"Oh, you'll see it."

"Well, probably not until I get there," I replied.

"True, but then you will know the tree."

Believe it or not, I could usually find their home. Just so you know, I found the tree.

Goals:

- No emergencies are caused or complicated by an inability to identify an address.

Interventions:

- Be sure that the address number outside the residence is easily visible to someone in a vehicle passing by it.
- Be sure the numbers are a distinctive contrasting color in comparison to the color behind the numbers.
  - o If the numbers are black, the post or garage door they are on is white.
  - o If the numbers are gold, the garage or post color is dark brown.
- Many homes have posts with address numbers located at the end of the driveway.
  - o This provides continuity of address location for the entire neighborhood.
- Sometimes people choose ornate signage for the address numbers.
  - o Script lettering for numerical addresses are not quickly identifiable.
- If numbers are placed directly on the house, be sure that trees or other structures don't block the numbers from being seen from the street or road.
- If the only house number is on the house and not at the end of the driveway, but sure the number is lighted at night in case an ambulance is trying to locate your home.

- **If your address number is on your mail box, be sure it is visible to those driving past.**
  - o **Be sure the number is on both sides of the mail box.**
  - o **You would not want an emergency vehicle to drive past your home, turn around, and then drive back because the number is only on one side of the mail box.**

SUMMARY:

Go outside and look at the house. If you did not know what the address number is, could you find it easily even it was dark? If not, see suggestions listed above.

Beerman, S., Rapport-Musson, J. (2002). *Eldercare 911*. Amherst, N.Y.: Prometheus Books.

National Institute on Aging. (2007). *So Far Away: Twenty Questions for Long-distance Caregivers*. (NIH Publication No: 05-5496). Washington, DC: U. S. Government Printing Office.

National Institute on Aging. (2012). *There's No Place Like Home – For Growing Old: Tips from the National Institute on Aging*. Washington, DC: U. S. Government Printing Office.

Chapter 42

AREA OF THE HOUSE . . . .
ENTERING

Potential Safety issues:

- **Falls.**

- **When emergency personnel need to enter your home and it is not clear where they are expected to enter.**

    o **This could slow down their potential response time.**

Just a thought:

Many times I arrived at a home in the middle of winter. Then it became obvious that the people living in the house only entered and exited through the garage. Sitting in a driveway, looking around, all I would see were mounds of snow on all the walkways around the house. The garage door was closed.

Whenever, there was a small door to one side of the large garage door, I would try to see if that were a potential entrance opportunity.

After knocking and waiting for several minutes, I would get back in my car and call on my cell phone. Several times they sounded surprised I was there.

"Why didn't you let us know you were here?" they inquired.

"How?" I wondered.

Goals:

- **Be sure if emergency vehicles were coming to your home, they could readily identify which door you expect them to enter.**

- **During snow seasons, be sure you have an emergency exit to allow more than one way out of the house.**

Interventions:

- **Walk around the outside of your house and identify ways that would be the most feasible means of entry if an ambulance or rescue car was needed.**

- **If you need assistance maintaining open sidewalks in case of emergency, consider hiring the service to be done routinely.**

- **Consider installing a doorbell outside a garage door, if that is your main entranceway.**

- **If you call for an ambulance be sure they are informed what to expect when they arrive.**

  - **This is helpful in case there is not an obvious front door; if they need an alternate entrance for their equipment, they need to know.**

SUMMARY:

Decide to visit yourself. Leave. Come back. Pretend you have never been at your own home before. By doing this, you could answer your own questions.

Beerman, S., Rapport-Musson, J. (2002). *Eldercare 911.* Amherst, N.Y.: Prometheus Books.

National Institute on Aging. (2007). *So Far Away: Twenty Questions for Long-distance Caregivers.* (NIH Publication No: 05-5496). Washington, DC: U. S. Government Printing Office.

National Institute on Aging. (2012). *There's No Place Like Home – For Growing Old: Tips from the National Institute on Aging.* Washington, DC: U. S. Government Printing Office.

Chapter 43

AREA OF THE HOUSE . . . .
STEPPING INTO THE HOUSE

Potential Safety issues:

- **Falls.**

Just a thought:

When I first entered homes, I never knew exactly what to expect once inside. Sometimes, there were amazing ornate entranceways. Other times, there were piles of shoes. At times, there was a designated carpet for placing your shoes and coat. Then there were other places where there was linoleum, so slick as to invite slipping even before anyone got through the door.

But the most challenging times were the dog owners with gates for keeping their pets corralled in specific places inside their home. Sometimes there were gates just inside the door in an attempt to keep pets inside. However, this was not always successful and they bounded out the door as soon as it was opened.

I respect the fact that an individual has the right to arrange the home the way they choose. However, when considering the older population, the percentage of falls that occur due slippery surfaces, clutter, or pets is significant. The thing to remember is that those could be preventable circumstances.

Goals:

- **No falls.**

Interventions:

- **Be sure that the entranceway is not wet or slippery.**
- **Remove clutter.**
- **Be sure that a person can enter the house completely, without fear of animals causing falls.**
- **Be sure that a person can enter the house completely, without fear of harm to any pets.**

SUMMARY:

Take a moment to re-evaluate your own home entrance. If there are items that could be placed elsewhere to provide a safer entrance, consider other options. Ask yourself, "Does it look like anyone could fall here?"

Beerman, S., Rapport-Musson, J. (2002). *Eldercare 911*. Amherst, N.Y.: Prometheus Books.

National Institute on Aging. (2007). *So Far Away: Twenty Questions for Long-distance Caregivers*. (NIH Publication No: 05-5496). Washington, DC: U. S. Government Printing Office.

National Institute on Aging. (2012). *There's No Place Like Home – For Growing Old: Tips from the National Institute on Aging*. Washington, DC: U. S. Government Printing Office.

Chapter 44

AREA OF THE HOUSE . . . .
LIVING ROOM

Potential Safety issues:

- **Falls.**
- **General Safety.**

Just a thought:

There have been living rooms in which I had the privilege of appreciating ornate decor with elaborate furnishings. Then there were other living rooms that needed help.

Some homes had more than one area for socializing. Then other places had one room used for cooking, eating, and watching television.

The variety of options for a living room is not the issue, but safety and a place to enjoy daily moments can give a living room the opportunity to be a very important place in the whole house.

Goals:

- **No falls.**
- **No fire hazards.**

- Adequate place to socialize.
- No general safety problems.

Interventions:

- Loose rugs need to be tacked down or removed.
- If people feel light headed when they stand up, consider where they might hit or might land on if they fall.
- Remove any coffee tables or decorative tables with sharp corners that could injure someone if they fall.
- Be sure all clutter is removed to avoid tripping.
- If hoarding is an issue refer to Chapter 30.

SUMMARY:

The living room could be a place to enhance quality of life by having a pleasant place to socialize. Evaluating potential hazards can help maintain and protect an individual's independence and dignity.

Beerman, S., Rapport-Musson, J. (2002). *Eldercare 911*. Amherst, N.Y.: Prometheus Books.

National Institute on Aging. (2007). *So Far Away: Twenty Questions for Long-distance Caregivers*. (NIH Publication No: 05-5496). Washington, DC: U. S. Government Printing Office.

National Institute on Aging. (2012). *There's No Place Like Home – For Growing Old: Tips from the National Institute on Aging*. Washington, DC: U. S. Government Printing Office.

Robinson, A., White, L., Spencer, B. (2007) *Understanding Difficult Behaviors*. Ypsilanti, Michigan: Eastern Michigan University.

Chapter 45

AREA OF THE HOUSE . . . .
DINING ROOM

Potential Safety issues:

- **Inadequate lighting.**
- **Inadequate space for people with walkers or wheel chairs to move around the room.**
- **Cluttered items may cause tripping or falls.**
- **Chairs that may not be optimal height for an older person.**
- **Loose rugs may cause falls.**

Just a thought:

Dining rooms are used for a number of different functions. Collecting the daily mail and sorting bills. Decorating the room with a sizable center piece. Placing shoes or items to be out of the way, but handy. Oh, yes, sometimes people eat at their dining room table.

Whatever the use, safety needs to be remembered. Carrying food and table settings back and forth from the kitchen need to allow for safety. In addition, all the furniture around the table is potentially helpful, or possibly a safety hazard.

Everyone has their purpose for the dining room. The safety issues are also unique based on the use of room.

Goals:

- **No falls.**

- **Optimal chair height for meals and socializing during meals.**

Interventions:

- **Be sure that there is no clutter to cause falls when walking around the table.**

- **Have cushions available for individuals to sit on to help adjust their height at the table.**

- **Be sure lighting is adequate during meals for individuals who may be visually impaired.**
  - o **However, be sensitive to issues of glare for anyone with Glaucoma.**
  - o **Challenges with vision may prohibit optimal nutrition.**

SUMMARY:

Periodically, take a walk around the dining room. If you cannot, then I suggest you take care of the items that need to be removed. Also, observe people as they are eating to be sure they can see and reach food easily.

Beerman, S., Rapport-Musson, J. (2002). *Eldercare 911.* Amherst, N.Y.: Prometheus Books.

National Institute on Aging. (2007). *So Far Away: Twenty Questions for Long-distance Caregivers.* (NIH Publication No: 05-5496). Washington, DC: U. S. Government Printing Office.

National Institute on Aging. (2012). *There's No Place Like Home – For Growing Old: Tips from the National Institute on Aging.* Washington, DC: U. S. Government Printing Office.

Chapter 46

AREA OF THE HOUSE . . . . OFFICE AREA FOR FINANCIAL PAPERS AND MAIL

Potential Safety issues:

- **Bills not paid timely.**
- **Potential fraud issues without realizing it.**
- **Not being able to locate papers when you need them.**
- **Missing important information needed for medical appointments.**
- **Clutter.**

Just a thought:

Another topic I heard all too often was, "We don't know where the money went." People who thought they were set for retirement suddenly realized that money wasn't there any longer.

At the same time, I have seen piles of statements in no particular order encompass the table, the sofa, the kitchen counter, and even the floor.

As people get older, trying to decipher the content of medical statements can be daunting. For some people who have never had experience on computers who are now trying to understand how to handle their finances electronically, the world of finance can become a whole new environment.

More than a few times, I was requested to explain health care billing statements. Knowing that I could only help them that one time while I was there, concerned me. Who would be there to assure that their money stays with them, and they would have their questions clarified?

Goals:

- **No Clutter.**
- **Organized bill payment system to prevent losing services.**
- **Forms needed for medical or legal reasons readily available.**
- **No fraud incidents.**

Interventions:

- **Prepare life decision documents before you need them.**
- **Have Durable Power of Attorney documents for medical and legal decision making completed soon and not during a crisis.**
  - o **Be sure to keep copies of the documents in a secure place.**
  - o **Be sure all individuals involved have pertinent copies.**
- **If someone has challenges remembering to pay bills, be sure that supervision is provided.**
- **Many banking institutions have fraud alert systems in place. It may be helpful to contact yours to find out what services they offer.**
- **Assure that bills do not get paid twice inadvertently by maintaining a current filling system.**
- **Request junk mail to stop.**
- **Consider having an adult child's name on the parent's account in case payments need to be handled on an urgent basis.**

SUMMARY:

Preventing financial dilemmas is less complicated and costly than trying to solve problems after they happen.

Beerman, S., Rapport-Musson, J. (2002). *Eldercare 911.* Amherst, N.Y.: Prometheus Books.

National Institute on Aging. (2007). *So Far Away: Twenty Questions for Long-distance Caregivers.* (NIH Publication No: 05-5496). Washington, DC: U. S. Government Printing Office.

National Institute on Aging. (2012). *Age Page: Getting Your Affairs in Order.* Washington, DC: U. S. Government Printing Office.

National Institute on Aging. (2012). *There's No Place Like Home – For Growing Old: Tips from the National Institute on Aging.* Washington, DC: U. S. Government Printing Office.

National Institute on Aging. (2013). *Legal and Financial Planning for People with Alzheimer's Disease.* (NIH Publication No. 08-6422). Washington, DC: U.S. Government Printing Office.

National Institute on Aging. (2014) *Advance Care Planning: Tips from the National Institute on Aging.* Washington, DC: U. S. Government Printing Office.

Chapter 47

AREA OF THE HOUSE . . . .
KITCHEN

Potential Safety issues:

- **Cleanliness/sanitation.**

- **Falls.**

- **Potential fire hazards.**

- **Difficulty preparing meals due to how items are arranged.**

Just a thought:

More than once I sat down at a patient's kitchen table. Then as I was ready to leave, the chart I was taking notes in, was stuck to the table. What seemed most interesting was that in each instance, the person standing there didn't react surprised.

The opposite type of kitchen was at times more of a concern to me. Sometimes I came into a home with two elderly people who didn't demonstrate much ability to take care of themselves, but the kitchen was spotless. It always made me wonder if they even cooked . . . or ate anything?

The kitchen can tell many stories about the people. What their priorities are. Whether their social habits include cocktails. Diabetics who can recite exactly what they are not supposed to eat, but their kitchen is full of high sugar pastries.

Goals:

- **No falls.**

- **No illness due to ingesting spoiled food.**

- **Kitchen is arranged to promote easy access to cooking utensils and food items.**

- **No fires.**

- **No injuries.**

Interventions:

- **Be sure any rugs don't slide.**

    o **Remove loose rugs from the kitchen.**

- **If a person is visually impaired or has memory issues, someone other than that person needs to be responsible for checking dates on refrigerated foods.**

- **Be sure to also check the freezer for out dated food items.**

- **It may be helpful to have an occupational therapist evaluate the way the kitchen is arranged.**

    o **Someone with training would be able to assist a person to maintain their highest level of safe independence.**

- **If there is any concern that someone may leave a stove burner on, consider removing the knobs from the stove.**

- **If a person has difficulty with maintaining clean surfaces, consider providing or hiring a service to be sure that there are no potential health concerns.**

SUMMARY:

For an older individual or couple, it is worth their dignity and independence to assist with a periodic assessment of how the kitchen appears. If a person demonstrates vision or memory deficits consider "helping" with a meal to see how they are doing. Sharing a meal could also help to determine if they need additional supervision.

Beerman, S., Rapport-Musson, J. (2002). *Eldercare 911*. Amherst, N.Y.: Prometheus Books.

National Institute on Aging. (2007). *So Far Away: Twenty Questions for Long-distance Caregivers*. (NIH Publication No: 05-5496). Washington, DC: U. S. Government Printing Office.

National Institute on Aging. (2012). *There's No Place Like Home – For Growing Old: Tips from the National Institute on Aging*. Washington, DC: U. S. Government Printing Office.

Chapter 48

AREA OF THE HOUSE . . . .
BEDROOM

Potential Safety issues:

- **Falls due to tripping over items on the floor.**
- **Falls due to inadequate lighting, especially at night.**
- **Falls due to falling out of bed.**
- **Head injuries due to falling onto furniture with sharp corners, e.g. dressers, bedside tables, etc.**

Just a thought:

I have seen many bedroom arrangements during my years as a nurse. Most homes had a bathroom close to the bedroom to make nightly trips to the toilet easy to do.

However, when bedrooms are down the hall or upstairs from the nearest bathroom, then additional safety issues present themselves. Making sure that rest and personal needs can readily be met needs to be a priority.

Goals:

- No falls for any reason.

- Appropriate lighting for when a person needs to get up during the night.

Interventions:

- Be sure the path from the bed to the bathroom is free of clutter.

- Obtain a nightlight or leave a light on in the hall or bathroom for night time.

- If there is furniture within three to six feet of the bed, place soft cushion type cloths over the corners or edges. In case of a fall, this could decrease the chance of lacerations to the head or scalp.

- Refer to Chapter 4 for directions how to prevent falling out of bed.

SUMMARY:

Be sure to look around the bed to visualize potential causes for falls. If there are shoes and other items located near the bed, help to determine an alternate location. Be sure to turn the lights off to assess whether night time lighting does not cause shadows that cause an increase in the chance of falls. Is the lighting adequate?

Beerman, S., Rapport-Musson, J. (2002). *Eldercare 911*. Amherst, N.Y.: Prometheus Books.

National Institute on Aging. (2007). *So Far Away: Twenty Questions for Long-distance Caregivers.* (NIH Publication No: 05-5496). Washington, DC: U. S. Government Printing Office.

National Institute on Aging. (2012). *Age Page: Falls and Fractures.* Washington, DC: U. S. Government Printing Office.

National Institute on Aging. (2012). *There's No Place Like Home – For Growing Old: Tips from the National Institute on Aging.* Washington, DC: U. S. Government Printing Office.

Chapter 49

AREA OF THE HOUSE . . . .
CLOSETS

Potential Safety issues:

- **Safety concerns regarding avoidable injuries.**
- **The unknown contents in a closet.**

Just a thought:

Closets are not usually a part of a typical home evaluation that I conducted as a geriatric nurse. However, closets present hazards for a number of reasons.

First, it is a potential concern if a person is living alone. If an elderly person tries to empty a closet and gets hurt, they may not be able to call for help. This has happened more than once to my knowledge.

Also, depending on what is stored, there may be items that families want to discuss and share. Cleaning out closets together could provide more of a meaningful time than a chore.

Goals:

- **No injuries.**
- **Preparation in advance if someone needs to move to an alternative living environment.**

Interventions:

- It is usually best to set aside time to work together to clean out closets.

- Agree on a plan regarding what items to keep, what to recycle, what to donate, etc.

- Do not assume that when someone with memory problems makes a promise that they will remember not to clean out the closet alone.

- Cleaning together can provide a time to reminisce about items found that bring back fond family memories.

  o Turn the "project" into a family event.

- During cleaning, be aware of structures inside the closet that may cause injury during the process.

SUMMARY:

It is wise to note that if a person lives alone family members should not assume they know exactly what their loved one is doing while no one else is around. If an idea causes someone to hunt for an object for whatever reason, unsafe decisions may take place. This may include going upstairs to clean out "storage rooms." Many adult children have told me they are sure their parent, "never goes upstairs when I'm not there." Are you sure?

Beerman, S., Rapport-Musson, J. (2002). *Eldercare 911*. Amherst, N.Y.: Prometheus Books.

National Institute on Aging. (2007). *So Far Away: Twenty Questions for Long-distance Caregivers*. (NIH Publication No: 05-5496). Washington, DC: U. S. Government Printing Office.

National Institute on Aging. (2012). *There's No Place Like Home – For Growing Old: Tips from the National Institute on Aging*. Washington, DC: U. S. Government Printing Office.

National Institutes of Health. (2010). *Caregiver Guide: Tips for Caregivers of People with Alzheimer's Disease*. (NIH Publication No. 01-4013). Washington, DC: U. S. Government Printing Office.

Robinson, A., White, L., Spencer, B. (2007) *Understanding Difficult Behaviors*. Ypsilanti, Michigan: Eastern Michigan University.

Chapter 50

AREA OF THE HOUSE . . . .
CLUTTER IN GENERAL

Potential Safety issues:

- **Falls.**
- **Fire safety.**
- **Emergency exit safety.**
- **Health safety due to potential for infectious environments.**

Just a thought:

There are a number of homes I could describe that I encountered during my years as a geriatric nurse where I was more than a little concerned about safety.

Sometimes, there was only a path to walk between the isles of shoes and clothes. Other times, the chairs needed to have their content moved to provide room for an extra person to sit down.

I know collecting can be a hobby, but when the items that have been collected obstruct routes to exits in case of a fire, then it becomes a problem.

Goals:

- **Cleanliness.**
- **Develop a plan how to achieve and maintain cleanliness.**

Interventions:

- **In the case where health and environmental safety is a concern, protective services need to be involved to assess the situation for vulnerable adults.**
- **Consider hiring a cleaning agency to tackle large potentially hazardous situations.**
- **If an elderly person or couple start to demonstrate an inability to maintain their home, act sooner than later before a crisis occurs.**
- **Always be sure there is more than one exit out of the house in case of a fire.**
- **Be aware that clutter may hinder emergency personnel from taking care of someone.**
- **Refer to Chapter 30 regarding hoarding.**

SUMMARY:

People have the right to choose how they live. However, if they become incapable of taking care of themselves or unable to determine safe decisions, family or other agencies may need to assume responsibility for that older person or couple.

Beerman, S., Rapport-Musson, J. (2002). *Eldercare 911.* Amherst, N.Y.: Prometheus Books.

National Institute on Aging. (2007). *So Far Away: Twenty Questions for Long-distance Caregivers.* (NIH Publication No: 05-5496). Washington, DC: U. S. Government Printing Office.

National Institute on Aging. (2012). *There's No Place Like Home – For Growing Old: Tips from the National Institute on Aging.* Washington, DC: U. S. Government Printing Office.

National Institutes of Health. (2010). *Caregiver Guide: Tips for Caregivers of People with Alzheimer's Disease.* (NIH Publication No. 01-4013). Washington, DC: U. S. Government Printing Office.

Robinson, A., White, L., Spencer, B. (2007) *Understanding Difficult Behaviors.* Ypsilanti, Michigan: Eastern Michigan University.

Chapter 51

AREA OF THE HOUSE . . . . BATHROOM

Potential Safety issues:

- **High risk of falls.**
- **High risk of injuries**.

Just a thought:

The bathroom, unfortunately, offers many opportunities for injuries. Not only is falling a concern, but there are more corners and objects to hit on the way down to the floor. Avoiding falls in the bathroom can prevent many injuries.

Getting in and out of the bath tub or shower is one place to be extra careful. When a person steps out of the tub, the foot that remains in the tub bears all their weight. When you transfer weight to your front foot from the foot that is still in the tub, that foot could easily slip and cause a person to lose their balance.

The reverse is true if you have a towel on the floor outside the tub. When one foot is on the towel and the other not, the towel acts like a banana peel in an old cartoon, except there is nothing humorous about falling in the bathroom.

One way to prevent falls getting in or out of the tub is to never use a towel. If you step on a rug or bath mat, be sure it has a nonskid surface on the bottom to avoid acting like a banana peel.

Goals:

- **No falls.**
- **No injuries.**
- **Sanitary surfaces.**

Interventions:

- **Remove all rugs that are not secure.**
- **Install grab bars.**
    - o **The best way to determine where to place grab bars is to stand in the tub or shower and observe where your hand would automatically go if you start to fall.**
    - o **Where your hand automatically grabs for something to hang onto, that is where the grab bar needs to be.**
- **Suction cup grab bars can be placed in any shower or tub. Remove and re-attach them once a month to be sure they are secure.**
- **Be aware of furniture that someone might hit if they fell after standing up from the toilet.**
    - o **Is there a sharp edge on the counter?**
    - o **Is there a shelf that a person's head could hit?**
    - o **Apply a cushion type cloth to any corner or edge that could cause an injury.**
- **Assess the lighting to be sure it is adequate if someone gets up to use the bathroom during the night.**
    - o **Sometimes it is too harsh to turn on room lights when a person has been sleeping.**
    - o **Softer bathroom lights or nightlights may be more practical.**
- **Do not stand on towels in the tub, shower, or outside of the tub or shower. A towel does not provide a nonskid surface.**

- If someone needs to have a rug outside of the tub, be sure to use a nonskid rug.

- Routinely sanitize all surfaces. For elderly individuals it may be helpful to consider hiring an agency for bathroom cleaning to assure thorough sanitation.

- Be advised that individuals who have glaucoma are usually sensitive to glare. Lighting in the bathroom may prohibit them from seeing areas that need to be cleaned.

- Also, people with macular degeneration may have visual field deficits that may cause that person to not see some problem areas.

SUMMARY:

The bathroom is potentially a high risk area for elderly people. When family members visit an elderly loved one, notice when you use the bathroom if there are odors or changes in the previous level cleanliness that their loved one had usually maintained. Also, be assertive about discussing how they are getting in and out of the tub and what they stand on when they first get out. Remember, grab bars cost less than a trip to the emergency room.

Beerman, S., Rapport-Musson, J. (2002). *Eldercare 911*. Amherst, N.Y.: Prometheus Books.

National Institute on Aging. (2007). *So Far Away: Twenty Questions for Long-distance Caregivers*. (NIH Publication No: 05-5496). Washington, DC: U. S. Government Printing Office.

National Institute on Aging. (2012). *Age Page: Falls and Fractures*. Washington, DC: U. S. Government Printing Office.

National Institute on Aging. (2012). *There's No Place Like Home – For Growing Old: Tips from the National Institute on Aging*. Washington, DC: U. S. Government Printing Office.

National Institutes of Health. (2010). *Caregiver Guide: Tips for Caregivers of People with Alzheimer's Disease*. (NIH Publication No. 01-4013). Washington, DC: U. S. Government Printing Office.

Robinson, A., White, L., Spencer, B. (2007) *Understanding Difficult Behaviors*. Ypsilanti, Michigan: Eastern Michigan University.

Chapter 52

AREA OF THE HOUSE . . . .
MEDICATION STORAGE

Potential Safety issues:

- **Not taking medications as prescribed.**
- **Taking medications more than prescribed.**

Just a thought:

One of the tasks I did when I visited patients for the Geriatric Assessment Clinic was to see where and how they stored their medications. Many times they would open a drawer or a cupboard and say, "Here they are."

As I scanned the mound of bottles I realized the dates on the containers varied from a few weeks to many years. I have no idea how many times I left the visit having no idea which medications they were actually taking.

When I would ask someone specifically how they knew whether they had taken their medications, I usually got the answer, "Oh, I have a system."

Actually, I think their system was the problem.

Goals:

- Take medications as directed.

- Knowing exactly what medications are being taken in case your primary health care provider needs to make adjustments in any of the medications or dosages.

Interventions:

- Always carry a list of all medications to all appointments.
  - o This needs to include prescription medications (the ones your doctor ordered)
  - o Plus, any over the counter medications or supplements you have decided to take based on your own information.

- Be sure to update the list every time there is a medication change.

- When medications are expired, get rid of them.

- Don't share medication from one person to another. Drug interactions may cause significant problems.

- It is always best to use a pill box to keep track of what pills are supposed to be taken each day and what time they are to be taken.

- If medication mistakes are noticed, be sure the primary health care provider knows before making adjustments.

- Keep a log of potential side effects to discuss at the next appointment.

- For additional information refer to Chapter 10.

SUMMARY:

Medications need to be taken as prescribed. If a clinician cannot tell what pills a patient is actually taking, then there is no way to know if the medications are effective. If dosages need to be adjusted, or consideration of whether a person is experiencing side effects, then an accountable person needs to verify what medications are actually being taken. This may mean that supervision of medication set up or administration is not negotiable.

Beerman, S., Rapport-Musson, J. (2002). *Eldercare 911.* Amherst, N.Y.: Prometheus Books.

National Institute on Aging. (2007). *So Far Away: Twenty Questions for Long-distance Caregivers.* (NIH Publication No: 05-5496). Washington, DC: U. S. Government Printing Office.

National Institute on Aging. (2012). *There's No Place Like Home – For Growing Old: Tips from the National Institute on Aging.* Washington, DC: U. S. Government Printing Office.

National Institutes of Health. (2010). *Caregiver Guide: Tips for Caregivers of People with Alzheimer's Disease.* (NIH Publication No. 01-4013). Washington, DC: U. S. Government Printing Office.

Chapter 53

AREA OF THE HOUSE . . . .
LAUNDRY ROOM

Potential Safety issues:

- **Falls due to clothing on the floor.**

- **Injury due to bending, stretching, twisting, or reaching when putting clothes in the washing machine or dryer or removing them.**

- **Inappropriate use of chemical substances.**

- **Potential injury due to "storage" not related to laundry.**

Just a thought:

With all the various challenges of having aging parents, it never ceased to amaze me when adult children taught me how to problem solve several concerns with one simple solution.

The best samples included moving the laundry facilities to the main floor. Sometimes they were able to relocate the washer and dryer into the bathroom. This saved their elderly parent effort and safety risks to accomplish staying clean.

Other times, the laundry was almost too convenient. It was a space readily available for storing everything other than soiled clothes. Perhaps the laundry room needed more cleaning than it provided.

Cleanliness was not only next to godliness, it can be very handy.

Goals:

- **No falls.**
- **No injuries.**
- **No clutter.**
- **Clean clothes.**

Interventions:

- **Due to physical limitations many elderly people find laundry of linen items to be very challenging.**
- **They may be able to take care of personal laundry, but then choose not to due to emotional reasons.**
- **Refer to Chapter 35 for further discussion about clothing.**
- **Be aware of all items in the laundry room.**
- **For people with memory issues, they may not remember what certain substances are intended for.**
    - o **Periodically, check what cleaning supplies are being stored and remove them if there is any chance they may not be used safely.**
    - o **Read labels for specific advice.**
- **Arrange the room so that clothing is never placed on the floor.**
    - o **This includes dirty as well as clean items.**
    - o **Dirty clothing provides a high risk for falls even if they are placed in the same vicinity.**

SUMMARY:

The laundry room is intended to aid in cleanliness. However, the safety concerns discussed above could actually cause this room to become a hazard.

Beerman, S., Rapport-Musson, J. (2002). *Eldercare 911.* Amherst, N.Y.: Prometheus Books.

National Institute on Aging. (2007). *So Far Away: Twenty Questions for Long-distance Caregivers.* (NIH Publication No: 05-5496). Washington, DC: U. S. Government Printing Office.

National Institute on Aging. (2012). *There's No Place Like Home – For Growing Old: Tips from the National Institute on Aging.* Washington, DC: U. S. Government Printing Office.

National Institutes of Health. (2010). *Caregiver Guide: Tips for Caregivers of People with Alzheimer's Disease.* (NIH Publication No. 01-4013). Washington, DC: U. S. Government Printing Office.

Chapter 54

AREA OF THE HOUSE . . . . CRAFT CORNER

Potential Safety issues:

- **Clutter.**
- **Small items like needles or pins on the floor and may not be seen by aging eyes.**
- **Various safety issues.**

Just a thought:

My grandmother sewed, knit, embroidered, tatted, and created various hand crafted items. Even as her hands crippled with arthritis and her vision narrowed by glaucoma, she still wanted to stay busy. She found a way to allow the sunshine coming in through the living room window to be her guide.

The sun doesn't stay in the same place all day. Neither did she. Sitting at one end of the room in the morning, she migrated with the rays of sunshine across the room. Like a cat warming itself in the sun moves to accommodate the cozy rays of the sun, Grandma would scoot her chair synchronizing her placement with the sun.

Goals:

- **No Injuries.**
- **Continue to enjoy hobbies of choice.**

Interventions:

- **Be sure items are stored in secure containers. Items that fall to the floor may not be seen.**
- **Be sure lighting is adequate for the individual. Individuals with glaucoma need softer indirect lighting instead of bright light.**
  - o **Other people may need brighter lighting to be able to enjoy their hobbies.**
- **Be sure to provide access to hobbies that a person enjoyed previously.**
  - o **As people age sometimes they may surrender doing tasks they once enjoyed.**
  - o **Provide encouragement as needed.**

SUMMARY:

When I get older I want everyone who knows me to have a size J crochet hook and fuzzy, soft blue yarn available within three feet of me every time I sit down. Please note that I prefer soft lighting. Consider this concept for someone you know.

Beerman, S., Rapport-Musson, J. (2002). *Eldercare 911*. Amherst, N.Y.: Prometheus Books.

National Institute on Aging. (2007). *So Far Away: Twenty Questions for Long-distance Caregivers*. (NIH Publication No: 05-5496). Washington, DC: U. S. Government Printing Office.

National Institute on Aging. (2012). *There's No Place Like Home – For Growing Old: Tips from the National Institute on Aging*. Washington, DC: U. S. Government Printing Office.

National Institutes of Health. (2010). *Caregiver Guide: Tips for Caregivers of People with Alzheimer's Disease*. (NIH Publication No. 01-4013). Washington, DC: U. S. Government Printing Office.

Chapter 55

AREA OF THE HOUSE . . . .
BASEMENT

Potential Safety issues:

- **Potential falls due to the stairs.**

- **Potential falls due to weakness in the railings.**

- **Potential for accidents depending on what items are located in the basement.**

Just a thought:

I heard many adult children offer concern about their parents going to the basement and whether it was safe or not. There are actually two issues about "going to the basement." First, is there a sturdy railing to support them? Second, is the lighting adequate to be able see?

Actually, once a person starts talking about going downstairs, a whole range of questions steps forward. Probably the most basic question is, "Do they really need to go down the stairs?" If the laundry is down there, how do they transport their clothes? If there is a workshop in the basement, is it safe for them to use the tools?

The contents of the basement are definitely a subject in addition to the safety issues going up and down stairs.

Goals:

- No injuries for any reason.
- No falls for any reason.
- If a fall occurs, the person has access to call for help.

Interventions:

- Assure lighting is adequate on the stairs as well as in the basement.
- Do not leave any items on the stairs.
- Check hand railings to be sure they are secure.
- If there are power tools refer to Chapter 56.
- Refer to Chapter 8 regarding laundry if the washing machine and dryer are located in the basement.
- Be sure anyone going downstairs has a life alert system or a cell phone with them.
    - o Even if there is a phone in the basement, check to see if a person could reach the phone if they fell down the steps and couldn't get up.
- Be sure that clutter is not a hazard.
- If items are carried to the basement, be sure that the person carrying the items can see the steps on the way down.

SUMMARY:

If it is unsafe for an elderly person to go to the basement, consider blocking off the door or locking it to prevent them from going downstairs unsupervised. Also, do not assume that someone with a memory problem would remember not to go downstairs even if they promised not to go down.

Beerman, S., Rapport-Musson, J. (2002). *Eldercare 911*. Amherst, N.Y.: Prometheus Books.

Cowley, G. (2000). Alzheimer's Disease: Unlocking the Mystery. *Newsweek*. (January).

National Institute on Aging. (2007). *So Far Away: Twenty Questions for Long-distance Caregivers*. (NIH Publication No: 05-5496). Washington, DC: U. S. Government Printing Office.

National Institute on Aging. (2011) *Age Page: Aging and Your Eyes*. Washington, DC: U. S. Government Printing Office.

National Institute on Aging. (2012). *There's No Place Like Home – For Growing Old: Tips from the National Institute on Aging*. Washington, DC: U. S. Government Printing Office.

National Institute on Aging. (2014) *Age Page: Exercise and Physical Activity: Getting Fit for Life*. Washington, DC: U. S. Government Printing Office.

National Institutes of Health. (2010). *Caregiver Guide: Tips for Caregivers of People with Alzheimer's Disease*. (NIH Publication No. 01-4013). Washington, DC: U. S. Government Printing Office.

Parkinson's Disease. (2012). In NIH online publication: *Senior Health*. Retrieved from: http://nihseniorhealth.gov/parkinsonsdisease/whatisparkinsonsdisease/01.html.

Chapter 56

AREA OF THE HOUSE . . . .
POWER TOOLS

Potential Safety issues:

- **Injuries due to lack of safe usage.**
- **Injuries due to cognitive decline regarding how to use the tools.**

Just a thought:

Many "do it yourself-ers" have established their workshops over the years. The collection of tools and left over parts from projects from long ago frequently surround the workshop or garage.

As Alzheimer's Disease progresses, the ability to remember what items were used for, not to mention how to use them safely, tends to decline. The memories of fun times come flowing back by the scent of the workshop. When nothing is connected to an electrical source, a person can reminisce without inadvertently injuring themselves.

It may present the best of both worlds. The privilege of strolling around the workshop can provide a sense of satisfaction. At the same time, the family can have the peace of mind that they are safe.

Goals:

- No injuries.
- Enjoy being around hobbies that had been a part of an individual's life.

Interventions:

- Provide supervision to help determine whether a person is still capable of using power tools.
- It may be helpful for a person to have neuropsychological testing to identify if there are deficits in visual perception, processing information, or memory that may impede safe use of equipment.
- If someone is not capable of safely using the tools remove the items to prevent an individual from hurting themselves.
- Unplug electrical cords and disguise outlets by covering them.

SUMMARY:

Sometimes it is difficult to take privileges away from loved ones. But if avoidable accidents occur, it is important to remember who is responsible. Do not allow someone to injure themselves when you know they are taking unsafe risks.

Cowley, G. (2000). Alzheimer's Disease: Unlocking the Mystery. *Newsweek.* (January).

National Institute on Aging. (2007). *So Far Away: Twenty Questions for Long-distance Caregivers.* (NIH Publication No: 05-5496). Washington, DC: U. S. Government Printing Office.

National Institute on Aging. (2011) *Age Page: Aging and Your Eyes.* Washington, DC: U. S. Government Printing Office.

National Institute on Aging. (2012). *There's No Place Like Home – For Growing Old: Tips from the National Institute on Aging.* Washington, DC: U. S. Government Printing Office.

National Institutes of Health. (2010). *Caregiver Guide: Tips for Caregivers of People with Alzheimer's Disease.* (NIH Publication No. 01-4013). Washington, DC: U. S. Government Printing Office.

Chapter 57

Area of the House . . . .
DECK/PORCH

Potential Safety issues:

- **High potential for falls.**
- **Potential for splinters from railings.**
- **Potential tripping on steps due to poor depth perception.**
- **Walking on a slick surface increases likelihood of falls and injuries.**

Just a thought:

I never really appreciated what it would be like to walk up a set of three steps to a deck until one rainy day. It wasn't just rainy. The precipitation was turning to ice as soon as it hit the ground and the deck. I had been driving and needed help. So, I walked up to the nearest house. Attempting to climb three slippery steps was intimidating enough. However, I needed to take just a few more steps to the door. At that point I had nothing to hang on to.

When an older person has lost confidence in their balance, and their strength is declining, don't assume they can accomplish tasks they have done previously. Also, the need for independence may prevent a person from asking or even allowing a helping hand.

What you can do is gently distract them by saying, "I'm ready to wish for sunshine right now." As you are talking, provide the hands-on assistance that will prevent them from falling.

Goals:

- **No falls or injuries.**

Interventions:

- **Be aware of loose steps.**
- **Is the railing reachable and able to be grasped?**
  - o **A railing that allows a person to have the thumb and fingers wrapped around it provides the individual better security for preventing falling or tripping.**
  - o **Be sure there are no splinters on the railing. Prevention is less painful than removing a splinter.**
- **In autumn, leaves can cause decks to become slippery.**
- **In winter, use a gritty substance to provide traction on icy decks. Kitty litter can be a handy example.**
- **If someone uses a walker routinely, be sure they do not use the walker when trying to go up and down stairs.**
- **Use the railing instead. Have a person with secure balance stand on the lower step while assisting the person to descend porch stairs. Using a transfer belt may help to prevent falls.**

SUMMARY:

Before there is an accident, walk around to assure that deck is safe for everyone. Would it be beneficial to add railings?

National Institutes of Health. (2010). *Caregiver Guide: Tips for Caregivers of People with Alzheimer's Disease.* (NIH Publication No. 01-4013). Washington, DC: U. S. Government Printing Office.

National Institute on Aging. (2012). *There's No Place Like Home – For Growing Old: Tips from the National Institute on Aging.* Washington, DC: U. S. Government Printing Office.

National Institute on Aging. (2007). *So Far Away: Twenty Questions for Long-distance Caregivers.* (NIH Publication No: 05-5496). Washington, DC: U. S. Government Printing Office.

Chapter 58

AREA OF THE HOUSE . . . .
GARAGE

Potential Safety issues:

- **There may be more hazards in the garage than what may be obvious at first.**
- **Lighting.**
- **Excessive storage.**
- **Stray items may cause tripping.**
- **Familiar items that may no longer be safe for that individual.**

Just a thought:

A garage can become a collecting place for many things. Outdoor equipment, garden tools, items from when the children were younger, contribute to multiple choices to potentially trip over.

Sometimes saying goodbye to items that are no longer used is almost like bidding farewell to the family memories. Prioritizing what things might still be useful, and how things are stored can actually increase the potential size of the inside of a garage.

Memories are important, but safety needs a place to stand.

Goals:

- No injuries.
- Safe entrance and exits.

Interventions:

- Does the person still drive?
    - o If not, why is there a car there?
    - o Does the car need to be removed or disabled?
- Are there any items, e.g. toys, garden items, etc., that could cause tripping?
- Is the lighting adequate so that hidden items will not be a tripping hazard?
- Is there garbage collected that could cause a health concern?
- Has hoarding caused an unsafe collection of various items?
- Are there power tools?
    - o Are they available for someone to use who could not assure their own safety?
    - o If individuals enjoy being around power tools and there is no access to electricity or other means of hurting themselves, e.g. sharp tools, this may be a positive source of activities.
    - o Refer to Chapter 56.
- Is there a lawn mower? Can the person use the lawn mower safely? If not, storage in a place where it is not visible could be good suggestion.

SUMMARY:

Garages offer a variety of potential safety hazards. As this can be a busy part of your home, it is advisable to routinely look around to be sure there are no potential safety concerns.

National Institute on Aging. (2007). *So Far Away: Twenty Questions for Long-distance Caregivers.* (NIH Publication No: 05-5496). Washington, DC: U. S. Government Printing Office.

National Institute on Aging. (2011). *Age Page: Older Drivers.* Washington, DC: U. S. Government Printing Office.

National Institute on Aging. (2012). *There's No Place Like Home – For Growing Old: Tips from the National Institute on Aging.* Washington, DC: U. S. Government Printing Office.

National Institutes of Health. (2010). *Caregiver Guide: Tips for Caregivers of People with Alzheimer's Disease.* (NIH Publication No. 01-4013). Washington, DC: U. S. Government Printing Office.

Chapter 59

AREA OF THE HOUSE . . . .
ROOF TOPS AND GUTTERS

Potential Safety issues:

- **Falling off ladders.**

- **Falling from unsafe heights.**

- **Injuries to hands from inadequate protective equipment.**

Just a thought:

Perhaps no one would think it necessary to discuss the concerns about roof tops and cleaning out gutters when discussing elderly people. Well, this chapter is a direct result of more than a few individuals who were injured as a result of climbing on ladders.

A sense of pride and independence encompasses many aspects of a person's identity. Sometimes the appearance of a home matters greatly to a family. Other times that sense of 'I can do it myself' and there is 'no reason to pay someone for what I can do,' attitude prevails.

Unfortunately, pride and self-satisfaction prohibit a person from realizing limitations that occur with the aging process.

Goals:

- No injuries.

Interventions:

- Consider removing ladders from the property if an elderly person may not remember not to use it.

- Consider hiring someone to be sure outside tasks are accomplished safely.

SUMMARY:

Independent minded senior citizens usually have considerable spunk and a sense of responsibility. It is good to not take away their sense of accomplishment. However, their safety should not be a risk. If they can't realize their own safe limitations, then families need to intervene for them. Injuries that prevent a person from living in their own home, do not promote independence.

National Institute on Aging. (2007). *So Far Away: Twenty Questions for Long-distance Caregivers.* (NIH Publication No: 05-5496). Washington, DC: U. S. Government Printing Office.

National Institute on Aging. (2012). *There's No Place Like Home – For Growing Old: Tips from the National Institute on Aging.* Washington, DC: U. S. Government Printing Office.

National Institutes of Health. (2010). *Caregiver Guide: Tips for Caregivers of People with Alzheimer's Disease.* (NIH Publication No. 01-4013). Washington, DC: U. S. Government Printing Office.

Chapter 60

AREA OF THE HOUSE . . . . GARDENS, YARDS, LAWN MOWERS, ETC.

Potential Safety issues:

- Potential falls due to walking on uneven ground.
- Potential falls due to imbalance.
- Potential various injuries due to misusing equipment.

Just a thought:

One of the treats I enjoyed as the nurse for the Geriatric Assessment Clinic was making home visits. With the number of lakes in Northern Michigan, the location of many homes I visited looked like vacation advertisements.

Garden walkways, patio furniture set to look out on Lake Michigan, a collection of bird feeders strategically placed to invite a variety of fine feathered friends, enhanced my time visiting with the people I came to meet. I can't help but admit the number of times I made a note of how I wanted to improve my own garden based on the esthetic wonder of those visits.

When I commented on their beautiful foliage, many times people would tell me stories that included many fond family efforts and memories. Now during the "golden years" appreciating family venues can provide a personal treasure.

Goals:

- **No falls.**
- **No injuries.**
- **Enjoy being outside in the fresh air.**

Interventions:

- **If people are supposed to use canes or walkers be sure they always use these devices outside.**

- **Be aware of areas in the lawn where there may be holes or other less visible concerns, e.g. mounds due to moles, garden hoses, etc.**

- **If someone has issues driving, then using riding lawn mowers may also require supervision.**

- **Consider having lawn chairs or benches available near gardens so that elderly people can enjoy being outside, but be able to have a place to sit without having to walk very far.**

- **In hot weather, be careful that people are not outside for a long time without having fluids to drink.**

SUMMARY:

For people who are lifelong gardeners, spending time outside can be a refreshing benefit for their mood state. It can also promote socialization and family time.

Beerman, S., Rapport-Musson, J. (2002). *Eldercare 911*. Amherst, N.Y.: Prometheus Books.

National Institute on Aging. (2007). *So Far Away: Twenty Questions for Long-distance Caregivers*. (NIH Publication No: 05-5496). Washington, DC: U. S. Government Printing Office.

National Institute on Aging. (2011). *Age Page: Older Drivers*. Washington, DC: U. S. Government Printing Office.

National Institute on Aging. (2012). *There's No Place Like Home – For Growing Old: Tips from the National Institute on Aging.* Washington, DC: U. S. Government Printing Office.

National Institutes of Health. (2010). *Caregiver Guide: Tips for Caregivers of People with Alzheimer's Disease.* (NIH Publication No. 01-4013). Washington, DC: U. S. Government Printing Office.

RESOURCES

Robinson, A., White, L., Spencer, B. (2007) *Understanding Difficult Behaviors.* Ypsilanti, Michigan: Eastern Michigan University.

National Institutes of Health. (2010). *Caregiver Guide: Tips for Caregivers of People with Alzheimer's Disease.* (NIH Publication No. 01-4013). Washington, DC: U. S. Government Printing Office.

Parker, W. H., Parker, R., Rosenman, A. E. (2002). *The Incontinence Solution: Answers for Women for All Ages.* New York: Simon & Shuster.

National Institute on Aging. (2013). *Age Page: Urinary Incontinence.* Washington, DC: U. S. Government Printing Office.

National Institute on Aging. (2011). *Age Page: Older Drivers.* Washington, DC: U. S. Government Printing Office.

Beerman, S., Rapport-Musson, J. (2002). *Eldercare 911.* Amherst, N.Y.: Prometheus Books.

National Institutes of Health. (2012). *Alzheimer's Disease; Fact Sheet.* (NIH Publication No. 11- 6423). Washington, DC: U. S. Government Printing Office.

National Institute on Aging. (2012). *Age Page: Falls and Fractures.* Washington, DC: U. S. Government Printing Office.

National Institute on Aging. (2014) *Age Page: Exercise and Physical Activity: Getting Fit for Life.* Washington, DC: U. S. Government Printing Office.

National Institute on Aging. (2012) *Age Page: Arthritis Advice.* Washington, DC: U. S. Government Printing Office.

National Institutes of Health. (2013). *Age Page: Osteoporosis: The Bone Thief.* Washington, DC: U. S. Government Printing Office.

Parkinson's Disease. (2012). In NIH online publication: *Senior Health.* Retrieved from: http://nihseniorhealth.gov/parkinsonsdisease/whatisparkinsonsdisease/01.html.

National Institute on Aging. (2014) *Talking with Your Doctor: A Guide for Older People.* (NIH Publication No. 05-3452). Washington, DC: U.S. Government Printing Office

National Institute on Aging. (2007). *So Far Away: Twenty Questions for Long-distance Caregivers.* (NIH Publication No: 05-5496). Washington, DC: U. S. Government Printing Office.

National Institute on Aging. (2014). *Alzheimer's Disease Medications.* (NIH Publication No. 08- 3431). Washington, DC: U. S. Government Printing Office.

National Institute on Aging. (2012). *There's No Place Like Home – For Growing Old: Tips from the National Institute on Aging.* Washington, DC: U. S. Government Printing Office.

Cowley, G. (2000). Alzheimer's Disease: Unlocking the Mystery. *Newsweek.* (January).

National Institute on Aging. (2011) *Age Page: Aging and Your Eyes.* Washington, DC: U. S. Government Printing Office.

National Institute on Aging. (2013). *Age Page: Depression.* Washington, DC: U. S. Government Printing Office.

Kalb, C. (2000). Coping with the Darkness: Revolutionary new approaches in providing care are helping people with Alzheimer's stay active and feel productive. *Newsweek.* (January).

National Institutes of Health. (2014). *Lewy Body Dementia: Information for Patients, Families, and Professionals.* (NIH Publication 13-7907). Washington, DC: U. S. Government Printing Office.

National Institute on Aging. (2014) *Advance Care Planning: Tips from the National Institute on Aging.* Washington, DC: U. S. Government Printing Office.

National Institute on Aging. (2013). *Legal and Financial Planning for People with Alzheimer's Disease.* (NIH Publication No. 08-6422). Washington, DC: U.S. Government Printing Office.

National Institute on Aging. (2012). *Age Page: Getting Your Affairs in Order.* Washington, DC: U. S. Government Printing Office.

U. S. Department of Health and Human Services, National Institutes of Health. (2013). *Your Guide to Healthy Sleep*. (NIH Publication No. 11-5271.6) Washington, DC: U.S. Government Printing Office.

National Institute on Aging. (2012). *Age Page: A Good Night's Sleep*. Washington, DC: U. S. Government Printing Office.

National Institutes of Health. (2013). *What's on Your Plate: Smart Food Choices for Healthy Aging*. (Publication No. 11-7708). Washington, DC: U. S. Government Printing Office.

National Institute on Aging. (2014). *Age Page: Hallucinations, Delusions, and Paranoia: Alzheimer's Disease Caregiving Tips*. Washington, DC: U. S. Government Printing Office.

National Institutes of Health. (2014). *Frontotemporal Disorders: Information for Patients, Families, and Caregivers*. (NIH Publication No. 14-6361). Washington, DC: U. S. Government Printing Office.